# Social Science 2EL0

# TABLE OF CONTENTS & ACKNOWLEDGEMENTS

**Week 3**

**Week 4**

**Week 6**

# WEEK 1

SOC SCI 2ELO

The Conference Board of Canada

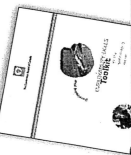

communicate, manage information, use numbers, work with others, be a

# Employability Skills 2000+

- Teamwork Skills
- Fundamental Skills
- Personal Management Skills

## Employability Skills 2000+

*The skills YOU need to enter, stay in, and progress in the world of work—whether you work on your own or as part of a team*

*Employability Skills 2000+ are the employability skills, attitudes and behaviours that you need to participate and progress in today's dynamic world of work.*

*The Conference Board invites and encourages students, teachers, parents, employers, labour, community leaders and governments to use Employability Skills 2000+ as a framework for dialogue and action. Understanding and applying these skills will help you enter, stay in, and progress in the world of work.*

---

## Member Organizations

Employability Skills 2000+ was developed by members of The Conference Board of Canada's Employability Skills Forum and the Business and Education Forum on Science, Technology and Mathematics.

AIESEC Canada Inc.
Alberta Human Resources and Employment
Alberta Learning
Association of Colleges of Applied Arts and Technology of Ontario
Association of Canadian Community Colleges
Automotive Parts Manufacturers' Association
Bank of Montreal
Bow Valley College
British Columbia Centre for Applied Academics
British Columbia Ministry of Education
Canada Post Corporation
Canadian Forces Recruiting Services Headquarters
Canadian Labour Force Development Board
Canadian Microelectronics Corporation
CAREERS: The Next Generation Foundation
Central Nova Industry Education Council
Conseil des écoles catholiques de langue française du Centre-Est — Ontario
CORCAN—Correctional Service Canada
Crain-Drummond Inc.
Dufferin-Peel Catholic District School Board—Ontario
Durham District School Board—Ontario
Elza Seregelyi and Associates, Inc.
Hewlett-Packard (Canada) Ltd.
Human Resources Development Canada
Imperial Oil Limited
Imperial Oil National Centre for Mathematics, Science and Technology Education
Industry Canada
Investors Group Inc.
J.D. Irving, Limited
Keyano College
Let's Talk Science
McGraw-Hill Ryerson Limited
Merck Frosst Canada & Co.
Mount Royal College
New Brunswick Department of Education
Nortel Networks
Ontario Ministry of Education
Ottawa Centre for Research and Innovation
Peace River South—School District No. 59—British Columbia
Peel District School Board—Ontario
Royal Bank of Canada
Saskatchewan Institute of Applied Science and Technology
Seneca College of Applied Arts and Technology
Shad International
Skills Canada—Ontario
Southwest Regional School Board—Nova Scotia
Statistics Canada
Syncrude Canada Ltd.
Software Human Resource Council Inc.
Toronto District School Board—Ontario
TransAlta Corporation
Treasury Board of Canada Secretariat
York University

Également disponible en français.
May 2000

---

## APPLY YOUR EMPLOYABILITY SKILLS AT WORK

Employability Skills 2000+ are the critical skills you need in the workplace—whether you are self-employed or working for others. Employability Skills 2000+ include communication, problem solving, positive attitudes and behaviours, adaptability, working with others, and science, technology and mathematics skills.

## APPLY YOUR EMPLOYABILITY SKILLS ELSEWHERE IN YOUR LIFE

Employability Skills 2000+ can also be applied beyond the workplace in your daily and personal activities.

## DEVELOP YOUR EMPLOYABILITY SKILLS

You can develop your Employability Skills 2000+ at home, at school, at work and in the community. Family, friends, teachers, neighbours, employers, co-workers, government, business and industry can all play a part in helping you build these skills.

## Looking for Ways to Improve Your Own Employability Skills?

**The *Employability Skills Toolkit for the Self-Managing Learner* Can Help You!**

The *Employability Skills Toolkit* is a suite of practical tools designed to help you:

- know yourself and get feedback;
- identify and reflect on your skills;
- plan skills development activities;
- implement your development plans and practise your skills; and
- document and market your skills for best success.

For more information on the *Toolkit* or how to work with the Conference Board to produce a customized version of the *Toolkit*, visit The Conference Board's Web site.

**www.conferenceboard.ca/education**

3

# Employability Skills 2000+

*The skills you need to enter, stay in, and progress in the world of work—whether you work on your own or as a part of a team.*

These skills can also be applied and used beyond the workplace in a range of daily activities.

---

## Fundamental Skills
The skills needed as a base for further development

## Personal Management Skills
The personal skills, attitudes and behaviours that drive one's potential for growth

## Teamwork Skills
The skills and attributes needed to contribute productively

---

*You will be better prepared to progress in the world of work when you can:*

### Communicate
- read and understand information presented in a variety of forms (e.g., words, graphs, charts, diagrams)
- write and speak so others pay attention and understand
- listen and ask questions to understand and appreciate the points of view of others
- share information using a range of information and communications technologies (e.g., voice, e-mail, computers)
- use relevant scientific, technological and mathematical knowledge and skills to explain or clarify ideas

### Manage Information
- locate, gather and organize information using appropriate technology and information systems
- access, analyze and apply knowledge and skills from various disciplines (e.g., the arts, languages, science, technology, mathematics, social sciences, and the humanities)

### Use Numbers
- decide what needs to be measured or calculated
- observe and record data using appropriate methods, tools and technology
- make estimates and verify calculations

### Think & Solve Problems
- assess situations and identify problems
- seek different points of view and evaluate them based on facts
- recognize the human, interpersonal, technical, scientific and mathematical dimensions of a problem
- identify the root cause of a problem
- be creative and innovative in exploring possible solutions
- readily use science, technology and mathematics as ways to think, gain and share knowledge, solve problems and make decisions
- evaluate solutions to make recommendations or decisions
- implement solutions
- check to see if a solution works, and act on opportunities for improvement

*You will be able to offer yourself greater possibilities for achievement when you can:*

### Demonstrate Positive Attitudes & Behaviours
- feel good about yourself and be confident
- deal with people, problems and situations with honesty, integrity and personal ethics
- recognize your own and other people's good efforts
- take care of your personal health
- show interest, initiative and effort

### Be Responsible
- set goals and priorities balancing work and personal life
- plan and manage time, money and other resources to achieve goals
- assess, weigh and manage risk
- be accountable for your actions and the actions of your group
- be socially responsible and contribute to your community

### Be Adaptable
- work independently or as a part of a team
- carry out multiple tasks or projects
- be innovative and resourceful: identify and suggest alternative ways to achieve goals and get the job done
- be open and respond constructively to change
- learn from your mistakes and accept feedback
- cope with uncertainty

### Learn Continuously
- be willing to continuously learn and grow
- assess personal strengths and areas for development
- set your own learning goals
- identify and access learning sources and opportunities
- plan for and achieve your learning goals

### Work Safely
- be aware of personal and group health and safety practices and procedures, and act in accordance with these

*You will be better prepared to add value to the outcomes of a task, project or team when you can:*

### Work with Others
- understand and work within the dynamics of a group
- ensure that a team's purpose and objectives are clear
- be flexible: respect, be open to and supportive of the thoughts, opinions and contributions of others in a group
- recognize and respect people's diversity, individual differences and perspectives
- accept and provide feedback in a constructive and considerate manner
- contribute to a team by sharing information and expertise
- lead or support when appropriate, motivating a group for high performance
- understand the role of conflict in a group to reach solutions
- manage and resolve conflict when appropriate

### Participate in Projects & Tasks
- plan, design or carry out a project or task from start to finish with well-defined objectives and outcomes
- develop a plan, seek feedback, test, revise and implement
- work to agreed quality standards and specifications
- select and use appropriate tools and technology for a task or project
- adapt to changing requirements and information
- continuously monitor the success of a project or task and identify ways to improve

The Conference Board of Canada

255 Smyth Road, Ottawa
ON  K1H 8M7 Canada
*Tel.* (613) 526-3280
*Fax* (613) 526-4857
*Internet*: www.conferenceboard.ca/education

# WEEK 2

SOC SCI 2ELO

# MY SKILLS LIST

This is not an exhaustive list.

| | |
|---|---|
| Accountable | Language |
| Accounting | Leadership |
| Adaptability | Listening |
| Administrative | Managing Projects |
| Analyzing | Mechanical |
| Artistic | Mediating |
| Athletic | Motivating |
| Attention to Detail | Multi-tasking |
| Assertive | Negotiating |
| Categorizing | Objective |
| Coaching | Observing |
| Computer Skills: (software, Internet, E-Mail) | Organizing |
| | Oral Communication |
| Confidence | Patience |
| Conceptualizing | Performing |
| Cooperative | Planning |
| Creativity | Positive Attitude |
| Critical Thinking | Presenting (Group Facilitation) |
| Customer Service/Focus | Problem Solving |
| Debating | Record Keeping |
| Decision-Making | Relationship Building |
| Dedication | Reliability |
| Delegating | Report Writing |
| Dependability | Research |
| Designing | Respectful |
| Determined | Responsible |
| Editing | Results-Oriented |
| Empathetic | Self-Motivated |
| Energetic | Selling |
| Evaluative | Sensitivity |
| Event Planning | Supervising |
| Flexibility | Supportive |
| Formulating | Teaching |
| Goal-Oriented | Teamwork |
| Hard Working | Time Management |
| Independent | Transcribing |
| Imaginative | Understanding |
| Insightful | Willingness to Learn |
| Interpersonal | Work Ethic |
| Interviewing | Written Communication |

SOC SCI 2EL0

# SKILLS WORKSHEET

This section is designed to help you identify the hard and/or soft skills you've developed through your prior experiences.
_Hard Skills_: skills that can be taught and then observed (e.g. computer skills, driving skills etc.)

_Soft Skills_: skills that are developed individually, and are difficult to be taught and observed (e.g. time management, organization skills etc.)

1. Think about your past & present work experiences:

| Where? | When? | What? (Responsibilities or Tasks) | The skills I learned or developed | |
|---|---|---|---|---|
| Hostess | High-School | · Positive Attitude at all times<br>· Clean the tables and seat people in an organized fashion | · Organization<br>· Time management | ☐ Hard skill   ☑ Soft skill |
| Sales Associate | High-School | · Interact w customers + help them find what they're looking for<br>· Hit a certain target of sales | · Computer skills<br>· Organization<br>· Dependability | ☑ Hard skill   ☑ Soft skill |
| Customer Service Rep | High-School + University | · Damage control<br>· Be able to firmly and politely decline<br>· Hit a target of resolved cases | · Written Communication<br>· Computer skills<br>· Organization<br>· Time management | ☑ Hard skill   ☑ Soft skill |

2. Think about your school experiences (high school, university, etc.):

| The subject/courses I enjoyed: | The skills I learned or developed | |
|---|---|---|
| Political Science | · Decision Making<br>· Debating + Delegating<br>· Written + Oral Com. | ☑ Hard skill   ☑ Soft skill |
| Sociology | · Written + Oral Com.<br>· Delegating + Debating<br>· Research + Report Writing | ☑ Hard skill   ☑ Soft skill |

SOC SCI 2ELO

3. Think about your volunteer experiences, your experiences with a team/committee or group:

| What was the experience? | Responsibilities or Tasks | The skills I learned or developed |
|---|---|---|
| Event Planning | · Coordinating the activities that would occur during the event<br>· Getting Special Permits | Computer skills · Planning<br>Written Com.<br>Record keeping / formulating<br>↗Hard skill   ↘Soft skill |
| Youth Counselor | · Coordinating activities<br>· Filling out forms<br>· First Aid + CPR/AED | · First Aid<br>· Planning<br>· Multi-tasking<br>· Negotiating<br>↗Hard skill   ↘Soft skill |

4. Complete these sentences:

a. People tell me I am good at:

Listening to a person's concerns and be able to help meet their requirements

b. A talent I identify in myself is:

Being able to analyze a situation and come up with different possibilities and/or outcomes

5. How will this exercise help me in my career? What are my transferable skills (soft skills)?

↳ Helps me identify the skills that I possess and that I could further develop

↳ My transferable skills are things such as :

· Planning
· Multi-tasking
· Goal - Oriented

SOC SCI 2ELO

10

# SAMPLE CAREER ACTION PLAN

**Careers I Am Considering...** (You must complete your action plan chart document found in AVENUE in full and upload to your PebblePad Portfolio).

Choose 3 occupations that are of interest to you and for each occupation, fill in: (1) "Why is this career a good fit for me?" and (2) "What are the potential disadvantages?"

| Occupation/Career Field | Why is this career a good fit for me? | What are the potential disadvantages? |
|---|---|---|
| Probation Officer | • I enjoy a job that has different tasks and challenges everyday<br>• I would like to work in an environment that provides a public service<br>• I have communication and interpersonal skills that would be useful in this career<br>• I would enjoy going to court and documenting cases | • High level of stress involved in this career<br>• Some work situations could pose potential threat to personal safety<br>• Would be difficult for me to keep emotions "at work" and not take them home at the end of the day |
| Researcher | • I enjoy thinking and analyzing information<br>• I enjoy working on my own when completing projects<br>• I would be happy to be able to contribute research findings to the greater community<br>• I would be able to present the results of my work at conferences and in front of large groups | • I sometimes have difficulty with statistical functions<br>• There is a higher level of education required and I am not sure I am ready to commit to this as of yet<br>• Although I enjoy working on my own, I also need some social interaction in my career |
| Event Planner | • I enjoy working with people<br>• I am able to organize and prioritize tasks effectively<br>• I enjoy planning and seeing the results of my work<br>• I feel that I would consider this type of work "fun" | • This involves a lot of work on weekends and in the evenings, and I am not sure that I would like doing that for an extended time<br>• This may involve managing/supervising others, and I do not have experience or a high skill level in this area<br>• I am not sure about the availability of jobs in this field |

## My Next Steps...

Choose one (1) occupation from the previous chart and include six (6) "Action Items" you can complete towards attaining this career.

You <u>must</u> complete **all 6 Action Items** and for each Item, indicate, "What will I gain?" and the "Date to be completed."

**Occupation: <u>Event Planner</u>**

| Action Item | What Will I Gain? | Date to be Completed |
|---|---|---|
| Attend the Continuing Education Fair | • To learn about post graduate education programs that may be suitable for me | October 2017 |
| Explore Career Cruising website | • To learn more about employability skills related to event planning<br>• To help me to think about where my skill "strengths" and "gaps" might be related to potential careers<br>• To find out about education required for this position | November 20-25 2017 |
| Google event planners in my area and contact them to conduct an information interview | • Gain practical insight into careers as well as advice on how to determine a good career path. (how to get my foot in the door)<br>• Networking opportunity (expand on possible future work opportunities) | January 2018 |
| Make an appointment to have my resume and cover letter critiqued at SSC | • To fine tune my application documents in preparation for applying to future positions | January 2018 |
| Search OSCARplus for job or volunteer opportunities | • Apply for positions/placements that would help me gain skills that are needed for event planning<br>• Focus job search on summer positions | January – April 2018 |
| Create a LinkedIn profile | • Connect with Event Planners to network<br>• Join planning discussion groups<br>• To find out about potential opportunities that exist | February 2018 |

**SOC SCI 2ELO**

# Job Posting: 54578 - Position: Beyond the Bell Educator

| | |
|---|---|
| **Application Deadline** | 09/15/2016 4:00 PM |
| **Application Method:** | OscarPlus |
| **Posting Goes Live:** | 09/14/2016 11:39 AM |
| **Job Posting Status:** | Expired |

## ORGANIZATION INFORMATION

| | |
|---|---|
| **Organization** | YMCA |
| **City** | Hamilton |
| **Province / State** | Ontario |
| **Country** | Canada |

## JOB POSTING INFORMATION

| | |
|---|---|
| **Position Type** | Part-time Internship |
| **Position Title** | Beyond the Bell Educator |
| **Position Location** | Various locations |

**Position Description**

**TO BE ELIGIBLE TO PARTICIPATE IN THE SOCIAL SCIENCES INTERNSHIP PROGRAM, STUDENTS MUST MEET THE FOLLOWING REQUIREMENTS** FROM THE TIME OF APPLICATION.
Students MUST:

- Be registered in 18 units or more in the Faculty of Social Sciences in a degree program for the Fall/Winter 2016/2017 session;
- Be in good academic standing with the university (not on academic probation);
- Be in good financial standing with the university (no outstanding financial accounts on the student record);
- Be registered in Level II or above (Please note that official registration for Level II begins only after the student has successfully completed Level I requirements and has commenced coursework for Level II, usually in September of their second year);
- Have completed SOC SCI 2EL0, Career Planning through Experiential Learning. No exemptions will be made; and
- All internship candidates must be authorized to work in Canada. International students must refer to the Government of Canada website http://www.cic.gc.ca/english/study/work-offcampus.asp to ensure eligibility before submitting an application.

**Please Note:** In addition to the eligibility criteria listed above, students must ensure that the internship placement is completed before academic requirements (formerly known as degree requirements) are fulfilled.

*APPLICATIONS WILL BE SCREENED FOR ELIGIBILITY BEFORE BEING PASSED ON TO THE EMPLOYER.*

SOCSCI 2EL0

**Organizational Overview:**

As one of the largest charitable community service organizations in Canada, the YMCA of Hamilton/Burlington/Brantford responds to critical social needs in the community and works to provide solutions. By nurturing the potential of children, youth and adults, the YMCA connects people to life-building opportunities, to each other and enhances their quality of life. We foster social responsibility and healthy living. The YMCA works collectively with community partners that share the YMCA's determination in strengthening the foundations of community for all people

This position requires a commitment to the YMCA mission and core values of: Responsibility, Honesty, Caring, and Respect, as well as, a commitment to building developmental assets in children and adults. All offers of employment will be subject to the provision that the successful incumbent provides the YMCA of Hamilton/Burlington/Brantford with a current and satisfactory Police Records Check. Positions responsible for the direct supervision of children and/or vulnerable persons will be required, in addition to a Police Records Check, to provide a Vulnerable Sector Screening Report at the time of hire.

**Nature & Scope:**

The Beyond the Bell Educator reports directly to the Beyond the Bell Supervisor. This position is responsible for the supervision of children, creating and facilitating the delivery of safe, age appropriate programming in an after-school program. The Educator is dedicated to improving children's academic competencies, values and physical well-being.

**Responsibilities:**
- Ensures safe, quality programs for participants and staff
- Collaborates with other staff, including the Supervisor, to ensure compliance of YMCA program standards
- Responsible for the completion and submission of weekly reports, evaluations and daily documentation with a focus on detail and accuracy
- Maintenance and evaluation of program equipment and materials
- Will identify problems and ensure issues are addressed by the appropriate manager/supervisor
- Models and complies with policies, procedures, best practices and employee expectations as established by the YMCA
- Works closely with the Beyond the Bell Supervisor ensuring program plans and activities are coordinated and meet the developmental and academic requirements of the program participants
- Available to work a regular schedule from 2:45 p.m. to 5:30p.m., however, is able to maintain flexibility in his/her schedule to manage issues, concerns and problems as they may arise
- Attends staff training and professional development activities as required

**Accessibility**

The YMCA of Hamilton/Burlington/Brantford is committed to creating an inclusive environment that accommodates all individuals, including those with disabilities. We support the goals of the *Accessibility for Ontarians with Disabilities Acts (AODA)* and have established policies, procedures and practices which adhere to the accessibility standards set out in the AODA. Should you require any accommodation throughout the recruitment process please do not hesitate contacting our Human Resources Department.

The YMCA of Hamilton/Burlington/Brantford is an equal opportunity employer.

## Position Requirements

### Qualifications:

- Post secondary education enrollment in a college or university program, preferably in child development and related fields
- 2 years experience working with children in direct program delivery
- Commitment to delivering programs for children
- Strong communication and problem solving skills
- Effective time management skills; must be able to plan and prioritize work assignments
- *Self motivated and able to work well independently and in a team environment*
- Knowledge of child development and related "new" research
- Ability to manage physical requirement of moving, unpacking and setting up program supplies and equipment on a regular basis

### Competencies:

**Commitment to Organization Vision and Values**
- Demonstrates and promotes a personal understanding of and appreciation for the Mission, Vision and Strategic Outcomes and Values of the YMCA.

**Communications**
- Communicates in a thorough, clear and timely manner and supports information sharing and goal achievements across the YMCA.

**Planning and Organizing**
- Establishes a clearly defined and effective course of action for self and others to accomplish short and long term work goals.

**Quality Focus**
- Ensures that success criteria for self, staff and programs are set, reviewed and surpassed regularly to provide excellent service delivery.

**Teamwork**
- Actively builds teams and encourages open relationships for maximum organizational effectiveness

SOCSCI 2EL0

| | |
|---|---|
| **All Degrees and Disciplines** | Yes |
| **Internship Work Schedule** | a regular schedule from 2:45 p.m. to 5:30p.m. |
| **Position Start Date** | September 2016 |
| **Position End Date** | June 2017 |
| **Duration** | 8 months |

## APPLICATION INFORMATION

| | |
|---|---|
| **Application Procedure** | OSCARplus |
| **Application Material Required** | Cover Letter |
| | Resume |

**Additional Application Information**

Please ensure that you are using simple fonts (i.e. Arial, Times) and that you PDF each document before uploading to OSCARplus. Be sure to double check your application package for any formatting errors.
**\*NOTE:** Employers may request students bring a copy of their official transcript to scheduled interviews. Please ensure to obtain copies of your transcript from the Registrar's Office or from the Faculty Office (KTH 129) as early as possible.

**If your application contains errors, omissions, or is of poor quality, it reflects negatively on you as well as the Experiential Education Office and will therefore NOT be passed on to the employer for consideration.**

*Students are not to contact the employer directly under any circumstances!*

SOCSCI 2EL0

# Job Posting: 60540 - Position: Crime Analyst Assistant

| | |
|---|---|
| **Application Deadline** | 02/03/2017 4:00 PM |
| **Application Method:** | OscarPlus |
| **Posting Goes Live:** | 01/25/2017 3:26 PM |
| **Job Posting Status:** | Expired |

## ORGANIZATION INFORMATION

| | |
|---|---|
| **Organization** | Peel Regional Police |
| **City** | Brampton |
| **Province / State** | Ontario |
| **Country** | Canada |

## JOB POSTING INFORMATION

| | |
|---|---|
| **Position Type** | Summer Internship |
| **Position Title** | Crime Analyst Assistant |
| **Position Location** | Brampton |
| **Salary** | Paid Internship |

**Position Description**

**TO BE ELIGIBLE TO PARTICIPATE IN THE SOCIAL SCIENCES INTERNSHIP PROGRAM, STUDENTS MUST MEET THE FOLLOWING REQUIREMENTS FROM THE TIME OF APPLICATION.**

Students MUST:

- Be registered in 18 units or more in the Faculty of Social Sciences in a degree program for the Fall/Winter 2016/2017 session;
- Be in good academic standing with the university (not on academic probation);
- Be in good financial standing with the university (no outstanding financial accounts on the student record);
- Be registered in Level II or above (Please note that official registration for Level II begins only after the student has successfully completed Level I requirements and has commenced coursework for Level II, usually in September of their second year);
- Have completed SOC SCI 2EL0, Career Planning through Experiential Learning. No exemptions will be made; and
- All internship candidates must be authorized to work in Canada. International students must refer to the Government of Canada website http://www.cic.gc.ca/english/study/work-offcampus.asp to ensure eligibility before submitting an application.

**Please Note:** In addition to the eligibility criteria listed above, students must ensure that the internship placement is completed before academic requirements (formerly known as degree requirements) are fulfilled.

*APPLICATIONS WILL BE SCREENED FOR ELIGIBILITY BEFORE BEING PASSED ON TO THE EMPLOYER*
SOCSCI 2EL0

17

The student will assist with the following :

- Data cleansing and compilation of crime data
- Data entry of modus operandi information into crime analysis database
- Reading and summarization of crime occurrences into database
- Sorting and filing of contact card information and related material
- Other duties as assigned

**Position Requirements**

- Preference to students in psychology/sociology or criminology
- High literacy in Microsoft Office Suite (Word, Excel, Access and PowerPoint)
- Detailed oriented and accurate data entry ability
- Strong interpersonal and communication skills

| | |
|---|---|
| **All Degrees and Disciplines** | Yes |
| **Number of Positions** | 1 |
| **Internship Work Schedule** | Monday-Friday |
| **Hours per Week** | 35 hours |
| **Position Start Date** | Monday May 1st, 2017 |
| **Position End Date** | Friday August 11th, 2017 |
| **Duration** | 4 months |

## APPLICATION INFORMATION

| | |
|---|---|
| **Application Procedure** | OSCARplus |
| **Application Material Required** | Cover Letter |
| | Resume |

**Additional Application Information**

Please ensure that you are using simple fonts (i.e. Arial, Times) and that you PDF each document before uploading to OSCARplus. Be sure to double check your application package for any formatting errors. *NOTE: Employers may request students bring a copy of their official transcript to scheduled interviews. Please ensure to obtain copies of your transcript from the Registrar's Office or from the Faculty Office (KTH 129) as early as possible.

**If your application contains errors, omissions, or is of poor quality, it reflects negatively on you as well as the Experiential Education Office and will therefore NOT be passed on to the employer for consideration.**

*Students are not to contact the employer directly under any circumstances*

SOCSCI 2EL0

# Job Posting: 60351 - Position: GIS Technician

| | |
|---|---|
| **Application Deadline** | 02/04/2017 4:00 PM |
| **Application Method:** | OscarPlus |
| **Posting Goes Live:** | 01/26/2017 2:36 PM |
| **Job Posting Status:** | Expired |

## ORGANIZATION INFORMATION

| | |
|---|---|
| **Organization** | Town of Saugeen Shores |
| **City** | Port Elgin |
| **Province / State** | Ontario |
| **Country** | Canada |

## JOB POSTING INFORMATION

| | |
|---|---|
| **Position Type** | Summer Internship |
| **Position Title** | GIS Technician |
| **Position Location** | Port Elgin, Ontario at the Municipal office |

**Position Description**

**TO BE ELIGIBLE TO PARTICIPATE IN THE SOCIAL SCIENCES INTERNSHIP PROGRAM, STUDENTS MUST MEET THE FOLLOWING REQUIREMENTS FROM THE TIME OF APPLICATION.**
Students MUST:

- Be registered in 18 units or more in the Faculty of Social Sciences in a degree program for the Fall/Winter 2016/2017 session;
- Be in good academic standing with the university (not on academic probation);
- Be in good financial standing with the university (no outstanding financial accounts on the student record);
- Be registered in Level II or above (Please note that official registration for Level II begins only after the student has successfully completed Level I requirements and has commenced coursework for Level II, usually in September of their second year);
- Have completed SOC SCI 2EL0, Career Planning through Experiential Learning. No exemptions will be made; and
- All internship candidates must be authorized to work in Canada. International students must refer to the Government of Canada website http://www.cic.gc.ca/english/study/work-offcampus.asp to ensure eligibility before submitting an application.

**Please Note:** In addition to the eligibility criteria listed above, students must ensure that the internship placement is completed before academic requirements (formerly known as degree requirements) are fulfilled.

*APPLICATIONS WILL BE SCREENED FOR ELIGIBILITY BEFORE BEING PASSED ON TO THE EMPLOYER.*

SOCSCI 2EL0

The successful candidate will assist the GIS Technologist and GIS Coordinator with several tasks including:
- GIS configuration
- GPS data collection
- Data Management
- Map creation

**Position Requirements**

- GIS knowledge necessary
- ArcGIS software knowledge necessary
- Good organisation skills, communication skills and attention to detail required

| | |
|---|---|
| **All Degrees and Disciplines** | Yes |
| **Number of Positions** | 1-2 |
| **Internship Work Schedule** | Monday to Friday |
| **Hours per Week** | 8:30am to 4:30pm |
| **Position Start Date** | May 1, 2017 |
| **Position End Date** | August 25, 2017 |
| **Duration** | 4 months |

## APPLICATION INFORMATION

| | |
|---|---|
| **Application Procedure** | OSCARplus |
| **Application Material Required** | Cover Letter |
| | Resume |
| | References |

**Additional Application Information**

Please ensure that you are using simple fonts (i.e. Arial, Times) and that you PDF each document before uploading to OSCARplus. Be sure to double check your application package for any formatting errors. **\*NOTE:** Employers may request students bring a copy of their official transcript to scheduled interviews. Please ensure to obtain copies of your transcript from the Registrar's Office or from the Faculty Office (KTH 129) as early as possible.

**If your application contains errors, omissions, or is of poor quality, it reflects negatively on you as well as the Experiential Education Office and will therefore NOT be passed on to the employer for consideration.**

*Students are not to contact the employer directly under any circumstances!*

SOCSCI 2EL0

# Job Posting: 61037 - Position: HR Intern

| | |
|---|---|
| **Application Deadline** | 02/26/2017 4:00 PM |
| **Application Method:** | OSCARplus |
| **Posting Goes Live:** | 02/05/2017 12:10 PM |
| **Job Posting Status:** | Expired |

## ORGANIZATION INFORMATION

| | |
|---|---|
| **Organization** | Fiat Chrysler Automobile (FCA) (formerly Chrysler Canada) |
| **City** | Windsor |
| **Province / State** | Ontario |
| **Country** | Canada |

## JOB POSTING INFORMATION

| | |
|---|---|
| **Position Type** | Summer Internship |
| **Position Title** | HR Intern |
| **Position Location** | Brampton Assembly Plant |
| **Salary** | Paid Internship |

**Position Description**

TO BE ELIGIBLE TO PARTICIPATE IN THE SOCIAL SCIENCES INTERNSHIP PROGRAM, STUDENTS MUST MEET THE FOLLOWING REQUIREMENTS FROM THE TIME OF APPLICATION.
Students MUST:

- Be registered in 18 units or more in the Faculty of Social Sciences in a degree program for the Fall/Winter 2016/2017   session;
- Be in good academic standing with the university (not on academic probation);
- Be in good financial standing with the university (no outstanding financial accounts on the student record);
- Be registered in Level II or above (Please note that official registration for Level II begins only after the student has successfully completed Level I requirements and has commenced coursework for Level II, usually in September of their second year);
- Have completed SOC SCI 2EL0, Career Planning through Experiential Learning.   No exemptions will be made; and
- All internship candidates must be authorized to work in Canada.   International students must refer to the Government of Canada website http://www.cic.gc.ca/english/study/work-offcampus.asp to ensure eligibility before submitting an application.

**Please Note:** In addition to the eligibility criteria listed above, students must ensure that the internship placement is completed before academic requirements (formerly known as degree requirements) are fulfilled.

*APPLICATIONS WILL BE SCREENED FOR ELIGIBILITY BEFORE BEING PASSED ON TO THE EMPLOYER.*
SOCSCI 2EL0

Fiat Chrysler Automobiles (FCA) US LLC, was formed in 2009 from a global strategic alliance with FIAT Group. The company produces vehicles and products under the Chrysler, Jeep®, Dodge, Ram, FIAT, SRT, and Mopar® brands. The combined resources, technology, distribution technology, brands, engineering, and manufacturing allow us to compete on a global scale. Our alliance allows us to build on the culture of innovation first established by Walter P. Chrysler in 1925 and FIAT's complimentary technology whose heritage dates back to 1899.

FCA takes great pride in fostering an inclusive work environment where employees can leverage strengths, experiences and perspectives. At FCA, we believe it is the diversity of talent and perspective that allows us to take a visionary approach, to strategically apply new technologies and forge ahead in our industry in innovation and performance.

**Job Description:**
The HR Intern is a temporary supporting role for the summer. The HR Intern will support hourly employment generalist duties, including the hiring of a full-time and part-time work force as well as completing transactions to ensure record integrity. Additionally the HR Intern would provide support to the training department.

Equal Opportunity Employer Minorities/Women/Protected Veterans/Disabled

**Position Requirements**

**Basic Qualifications:**
- Student (2nd year or above) in a University degreed program
- Computer experience is required (MS Excel, Word and Access)
- Strong interpersonal and communication skills
- Must be eligible to work in Canada

**Preferred Qualifications:**
- Previous experience creating databases

| | |
|---|---|
| **All Degrees and Disciplines** | Yes |
| **Number of Positions** | 1 |
| **Hours per Week** | Full-time |
| **Position Start Date** | TBD |
| **Position End Date** | TBD |
| **Duration** | 4 months |

SOCSCI 2EL0

# APPLICATION INFORMATION

**Application Procedure**          OSCARplus
**Application Material Required**  Cover Letter
                                  Resume
                                  Unofficial Transcript

**Additional Application Information**

**This is a two-step application process:**

1. Apply via OSCARplus
         Please reference Req# 1019755 on your cover letter
AND

2. To be considered, you MUST apply on the company website

Please ensure that you are using simple fonts (i.e. Arial, Times) and that you PDF each document before uploading to OSCARplus. Be sure to double check your application package for any formatting errors.
**\*NOTE:** Employers may request students bring a copy of their official transcript to scheduled interviews. Please ensure to obtain copies of your transcript from the Registrar's Office or from the Faculty Office (KTH 129) as early as possible.

**If your application contains errors, omissions, or is of poor quality, it reflects negatively on you as well as the Experiential Education Office and will therefore NOT be passed on to the employer for consideration.**

*Students are not to contact the employer directly under any circumstances!*

SOCSCI 2EL0

24

# Job Posting: 53806 - Position: Jr. Analyst, Socio-economic Information

| | |
|---|---|
| **Application Deadline** | 07/30/2016 4:00 PM |
| **Application Method:** | OSCARplus |
| **Posting Goes Live:** | 07/27/2016 11:17 PM |
| **Job Posting Status:** | Expired |

## ORGANIZATION INFORMATION

| | |
|---|---|
| **Organization** | Service Canada |
| **City** | Toronto |
| **Province / State** | Ontario |
| **Country** | Canada |

## JOB POSTING INFORMATION

| | |
|---|---|
| **Position Type** | Full-time Internship |
| **Position Title** | Jr. Analyst, Socio-economic Information |
| **Position Location** | Ontario Regional Headquarters, 4900 Yonge St., Toronto, ON, M2N 6A8 |
| **Salary** | Paid Internship |

**Position Description**

**TO BE ELIGIBLE TO PARTICIPATE IN THE SOCIAL SCIENCES INTERNSHIP PROGRAM, STUDENTS MUST MEET THE FOLLOWING REQUIREMENTS FROM THE TIME OF APPLICATION.** Students MUST:

- Registered in 18 units or more in the Faculty of Social Sciences in a degree program for the Fall/Winter 2016/2017 session;
- Be in good academic standing with the university (not on academic probation);
- Be in good financial standing with the university (no outstanding financial accounts on the student record);
- Be registered in Level II or above (Please note that official registration for Level II begins only after the student has successfully completed Level I requirements and has commenced coursework for Level II, usually in September of their second year);
- Have completed SOC SCI 2EL0, Career Planning through Experiential Learning.  No exemptions will be made; and
- All internship candidates must be authorized to work in Canada. International students must refer to the Government of Canada website http://www.cic.gc.ca/english/study/work-offcampus.asp to ensure eligibility before submitting an application.

**Please Note:** In addition to the eligibility criteria listed above, students must ensure that the internship placement is completed before degree requirements are fulfilled.

*APPLICATIONS WILL BE SCREENED FOR ELIGIBILITY BEFORE BEING PASSED ON TO THE EMPLOYER.*

SOCSCI 2EL0

**Overview:**

The Labour Market and Socio-economic Information Directorate (LMSID) is responsible for monitoring the Ontario labour market and researching, analysing and reporting on demographic and socio-economic trends within local communities. The information LMSID collects and analyses is used to support internal strategic decision-making related to the delivery of Service Canada's programs and services, as well as to inform Canadians on occupational, industrial and socio-economic trends affecting Ontario. The Co-op student will support LMSID by carrying out the activities summarized below.

KEY ACTIVITIES / JOB DUTIES:
- Track and report on labour market developments in select local communities
- Conduct and/or participate in research and analysis of socio-economic issues, demographic and labour market trends
- Maintain, extract and synthesise data from socio-economic, demographic and labour market information databases to respond to internal and external information requests. This may require the ability to use software programs such as Beyond 20/20, SAS, Eviews and Excel.
- Prepare occupational trend reports using both quantitative and qualitative data
- Assist in developing and delivering presentations on socio-economic and labour market information to users
- Assist in conducting socio-economic analysis using geographic mapping software

**Position Requirements**

**1. Education and Experience:**
- Student must be enrolled in their 3rd or 4th year of full-time studies in the Economics program at the selected university.

Note: To be eligible, students must be registered with their academic institution's Co-op and/or Internship program. Proof of this will be required prior to appointment.
- Experience in researching and analyzing labour market or socio-economic information is an asset, but is not required

**2. Knowledge and Abilities:**
- Knowledge of the labour market, and social issues and economic factors influencing labour market conditions
- Knowledge of research methods and quantitative and qualitative analysis, principles, tools and techniques
- Knowledge of statistical modelling principles, tools and techniques
- Communication – Oral
- Communication – Written

**3. Personal Suitability:**
- Dependability
- Working with others

SOCSCI 2EL0

OFFICIAL LANGUAGE PROFICIENCY:

- English essential

| | |
|---|---|
| **All Degrees and Disciplines** | Yes |
| **Number of Positions** | 1 |
| **Hours per Week** | 37.5 |
| **Position Start Date** | August 31, 2016 |
| **Position End Date** | December 18, 2016 |
| **Duration** | 4 months |

## APPLICATION INFORMATION

| | |
|---|---|
| **Application Procedure** | OSCARplus |
| **Application Material Required** | Cover Letter |
| | Resume |
| | Unofficial Transcript |

### Additional Application Information

Please ensure that you are using simple fonts (i.e. Arial, Times) and that you PDF each document before uploading to OSCARplus. Be sure to double check your application package for any formatting errors.
*NOTE: Employers may request students bring a copy of their official transcript to scheduled interviews. Please ensure to obtain copies of your transcript from the Registrar's Office or from the Faculty Office (KTH 129) as early as possible.

**If your application contains errors, omissions, or is of poor quality, it reflects negatively on you as well as the Experiential Education Office and will therefore NOT be passed on to the employer for consideration.**

*Students are not to contact the employer directly under any circumstances!*

SOCSCI 2EL0

# Job Posting: 62028 - Position: Policy Analyst

| | |
|---|---|
| **Application Deadline** | 03/10/2017 4:00 PM |
| **Application Method:** | OSCARplus |
| **Posting Goes Live:** | 03/02/2017 1:33 PM |
| **Job Posting Status:** | Expired |

## ORGANIZATION INFORMATION

| | |
|---|---|
| **Organization** | Government of Ontario |
| **City** | Toronto, ON |
| **Province / State** | Ontario |
| **Country** | Canada |

## JOB POSTING INFORMATION

| | |
|---|---|
| **Position Type** | Summer Internship |
| **Position Title** | Policy Analyst |
| **Position Location** | Toronto |
| **Salary** | Paid Internship |

### Position Description

**TO BE ELIGIBLE TO PARTICIPATE IN THE SOCIAL SCIENCES INTERNSHIP PROGRAM, STUDENTS MUST MEET THE FOLLOWING REQUIREMENTS <u>FROM THE TIME OF APPLICATION.</u>**
Students MUST:

- Be registered in 18 units or more in the Faculty of Social Sciences in a degree program for the Fall/Winter 2016/2017   session;
- Be in good academic standing with the university (not on academic probation);
- Be in good financial standing with the university (no outstanding financial accounts on the student record);
- Be registered in Level II or above (Please note that official registration for Level II begins only after the student has successfully completed Level I requirements and has commenced coursework for Level II, usually in September of their second year);
- Have completed SOC SCI 2EL0, Career Planning through Experiential Learning.   <u>No exemptions will be made;</u> and
- All internship candidates must be authorized to work in Canada.    International students must refer to the Government of Canada website <u>http://www.cic.gc.ca/english/study/work-offcampus.asp</u> to ensure eligibility before submitting an application.

**Please Note:** In addition to the eligibility criteria listed above, students must ensure that the internship placement is completed before academic requirements (formerly known as degree requirements) are fulfilled.

*APPLICATIONS WILL BE SCREENED FOR ELIGIBILITY BEFORE BEING PASSED ON TO THE EMPLOYER*
SOCSCI 2EL0

## Job Description Summary

The Commercialization branch leads the development and implementation of strategies and programs to ensure that robust commercialization services, such as access to capital, business acceleration services, industry-academic collaboration programs, mentoring, training and networking, are available to innovative companies, entrepreneurs and researchers across Ontario. The branch is divided into two units:

### 1) The Network Programs Unit

Supports the innovation focused components of the Ontario Network of Entrepreneurs (onebusiness.ca) specifically the Regional and Sector Innovation Centres, the Industry Academic Collaboration Program and the Business Acceleration Program. These programs together support the launch and growth of globally competitive technology-oriented companies, and leverage the province's research institutions through knowledge and technology transfer, and collaborative research activities.

### 2) The Capital Programs Unit

- Develops and delivers provincial programs to enable Ontario firms to scale up, build market presence and access growth capital. The unit supports commercialization opportunities at different stages of the innovation continuum.

### Responsibilities:

- Conduct research and analysis as requested and synthesize findings into briefing materials for Ministry executives, including the Minister;
- Plan and participate in industry meetings and events;
- Works with partners in other Ministries, external agencies, industry associations and companies to identify strategic issues, trends, competitive strengths/challenges in support of program/policy development.

### Position Requirements

### Required Skills:

- Research and analysis, organizational skills;
- Ability to produce deliverables within tight deadlines;
- Good written and oral communication skills;
- Work as part of a team, with strong interpersonal skills;
- Proficiency with word-processing, spreadsheet, database-management/development, presentation/other software; and,
- Ability to perform data/information searches, and preform data entry as needed.

SOCSCI 2EL0

| | |
|---|---|
| **All Degrees and Disciplines** | Yes |
| **Number of Positions** | 1 |
| **Hours per Week** | 36.25 hours per week |
| **Position Start Date** | May 1, 2017 |
| **Position End Date** | August 25, 2017 |
| **Duration** | 4 months |

## APPLICATION INFORMATION

| | |
|---|---|
| **Application Procedure** | OSCARplus |
| **Application Material Required** | Cover Letter |
| | Resume |
| | Unofficial Transcript |

**Additional Application Information**

**PLEASE BE SURE TO TAILOR YOUR COVER LETTER AND RESUME TO THE JOB POSTING.**

Please ensure that you are using simple fonts (i.e. Arial, Times) and that you PDF each document before uploading to OSCARplus. Be sure to double check your application package for any formatting errors.
*NOTE: Employers may request students bring a copy of their official transcript to scheduled interviews. Please ensure to obtain copies of your transcript from the Registrar's Office or from the Faculty Office (KTH 129) as early as possible.

**If your application contains errors, omissions, or is of poor quality, it reflects negatively on you as well as the Experiential Education Office and will therefore NOT be passed on to the employer for consideration.**

*Students are not to contact the employer directly under any circumstances!*

SOCSCI 2EL0

## Job Posting: 62316 - Position: Program Assistant, Focus on Youth Program

| | |
|---|---|
| **Application Deadline** | 03/29/2017 4:00 PM |
| **Application Method:** | OscarPlus |
| **Posting Goes Live:** | 03/11/2017 2:32 PM |
| **Job Posting Status:** | Expired |

## ORGANIZATION INFORMATION

| | |
|---|---|
| **Organization** | Hamilton-Wentworth District School Board |
| **City** | Hamilton |
| **Province / State** | Ontario |
| **Country** | Canada |

## JOB POSTING INFORMATION

| | |
|---|---|
| **Position Type** | Summer Internship |
| **Position Title** | Program Assistant, Focus on Youth Program |
| **Position Location** | Hamilton, ON |
| **Salary** | Paid Internship |

**Position Description**

**TO BE ELIGIBLE TO PARTICIPATE IN THE SOCIAL SCIENCES INTERNSHIP PROGRAM, STUDENTS MUST MEET THE FOLLOWING REQUIREMENTS FROM THE TIME OF APPLICATION.**
Students MUST:

- Be registered in 18 units or more in the Faculty of Social Sciences in a degree program for the Fall/Winter 2016/2017 session;
- Be in good academic standing with the university (not on academic probation);
- Be in good financial standing with the university (no outstanding financial accounts on the student record);
- Be registered in Level II or above (Please note that official registration for Level II begins only after the student has successfully completed Level I requirements and has commenced coursework for Level II, usually in September of their second year);
- Have completed SOC SCI 2EL0, Career Planning through Experiential Learning. No exemptions will be made; and
- All internship candidates must be authorized to work in Canada. International students must refer to the Government of Canada website http://www.cic.gc.ca/english/study/work-offcampus.asp to ensure eligibility before submitting an application.

**Please Note:** In addition to the eligibility criteria listed above, students must ensure that the internship placement is completed before academic requirements (formerly known as degree requirements) are fulfilled.

*APPLICATIONS WILL BE SCREENED FOR ELIGIBILITY BEFORE BEING PASSED ON TO THE EMPLOYER.*

SOCSCI 2EL0

**Summary of Duties:**

Under the direction of the HWDSB Community Engagement Specialist and working with the Student Leadership Development Lead responsible for the recruitment and hiring of student employees and student leadership development, the Program Assistant will provide support for the leadership, supervision, program planning and team building of the secondary students hired through the Focus on Youth program.

**General Duties:**
- Responsible for supporting the interviewing, hiring and program support of secondary students in multiple Focus on Youth program locations
- Responsible for promoting and attracting program participants for HWDSB and community agency summer programs
- Assists students in the successful performance of their duties in their programs including training, conducting meetings and monitoring attendance
- Acts as a mediator when issues or problems arise in student placements
- Prepares and submits all required administrative documents on the program and student employees
- Ensures that the policies and procedures of HWDSB are followed and maintained
- Ensures the safety of all students, while participating in the programs, by working in accordance with the provisions of applicable health and safety legislation and all HWDSB policies and procedures
- Performs other duties as assigned
- Please note that some evening work will be required as part of this position

**Position Requirements:**
- Currently enrolled in a post-secondary education program combined with related work experience working with children and youth
- Demonstrated experience supervising and leading youth
- Strong communication skills, both orally and in written form
- Must have excellent organizational and public relation skills
- Ability to lead consistently and provide objective evaluation
- Criminal Record Check (vulnerable sector) valid within 6 months
- Must have access to reliable transportation with the ability to respond to urgent needs across the district

| | |
|---|---|
| **All Degrees and Disciplines** | Yes |
| **Number of Positions** | 1 |
| **Hours per Week** | 35 hours |
| **Position Start Date** | Monday, April 17, 2017 |
| **Position End Date** | Friday, August 11, 2017 |
| **Duration** | 4 months |

SOCSCI 2EL0

# APPLICATION INFORMATION

**Application Procedure**    OSCARplus
**Application Material Required**    Cover Letter
                                      Resume

**Additional Application Information**

**PLEASE BE SURE TO TAILOR YOUR COVER LETTER AND RESUME TO THE JOB POSTING.**

Please ensure that you are using simple fonts (i.e. Arial, Times) and that you PDF each document before uploading to OSCARplus. Be sure to double check your application package for any formatting errors.
**\*NOTE:** Employers may request students bring a copy of their official transcript to scheduled interviews. Please ensure to obtain copies of your transcript from the Registrar's Office or from the Faculty Office (KTH 129) as early as possible.

**If your application contains errors, omissions, or is of poor quality, it reflects negatively on you as well as the Experiential Education Office and will therefore NOT be passed on to the employer for consideration.**

*Students are not to contact the employer directly under any circumstances!*

SOCSCI 2EL0

# Job Posting: 49909 - Position: Public Policy Intern

| | |
|---|---|
| **Application Deadline** | 04/09/2016 4:00 PM |
| **Application Method:** | OSCARplus |
| **Posting Goes Live:** | 04/02/2016 2:43 PM |
| **Job Posting Status:** | Expired |

## ORGANIZATION INFORMATION

| | |
|---|---|
| **Organization** | Hoffmann-La Roche Ltd. |
| **City** | Mississauga |
| **Province / State** | Ontario |
| **Country** | Canada |

## JOB POSTING INFORMATION

| | |
|---|---|
| **Position Type** | Full-time Internship |
| **Position Title** | Public Policy Intern |
| **Position Location** | Mississauga ON |

**Position Description**

**TO BE ELIGIBLE TO PARTICIPATE IN THE SOCIAL SCIENCES INTERNSHIP PROGRAM, STUDENTS MUST MEET THE FOLLOWING REQUIREMENTS   FROM THE TIME OF APPLICATION.**

Students MUST:
- Registered in 18 units or more in the Faculty of Social Sciences in a degree program for the Fall/Winter 2016/2017 session;
- Be in good academic standing with the university (not on academic probation);
- Be in good financial standing with the university (no outstanding financial accounts on the student record);
- Be registered in Level II or above (Please note that official registration for Level II begins only after the student has successfully completed Level I requirements and has commenced coursework for Level II, usually in September of their second year);
- Have completed SOC SCI 2EL0, Career Planning through Experiential Learning. <u>No exemptions will be made</u>; and
- All internship candidates must be authorized to work in Canada.  International students must refer to the Government of Canada website http://www.cic.gc.ca/english/study/work-offcampus.asp to ensure eligibility before submitting an application.

**Please Note:** In addition to the eligibility criteria listed above, students must ensure that the internship placement is completed before degree requirements are fulfilled.

*APPLICATIONS WILL BE SCREENED FOR ELIGIBILITY BEFORE BEING PASSED ON TO THE EMPLOYER.*

SOCSCI 2EL0

Company Information:

Hoffmann-La Roche Limited is a leading global healthcare company committed to the discovery and research of new and innovative medicines to treat human illnesses. The company is active in a broad range of therapeutic categories that include: oncology, hepatitis, infectious diseases, transplant, arthritis and metabolism.

Hoffmann-La Roche Limited is currently seeking one qualified student for the position of Health Policy Intern for our Canadian (pharmaceutical division) head office, located in Mississauga, ON.

Job description:

The responsibilities of the Public Policy Intern position are:

- Work with GR & Health Policy Managers, as well as cross functional teams, in the development of policy position papers pertaining to healthcare sustainability and other national public policy issues
- Providing regular updates and analysis on health and public policy news, trends, reports
- Development of an internal policy communications website and tools
- Coordination and delivery of action items from Policy team meetings
- Point person for liaison to various cross-functional units regarding project deliverables
- Arranging meetings and developing agendas/sending out minutes and action items
- Development of key documents and marshalling through approval process
- Development of core policy business review profile by province including investments, partnerships, product and pipeline overview
- Work with cross-functional teams on personalized healthcare and subsequent entry biologics policy
- Liaison with Government Relations team regarding provincial policy deliverables

**Position Requirements**

Skills/Experience Preferred:

- Health Studies, Government Affairs, Public Policy, Political Science, Economy, Social Sciences, Communications, Journalism or Life Sciences disciplines strongly preferred.
- Genuine interest in the health care industry
- Strong analytical and critical appraisal skills
- Excellent written and oral communication skills, proficiency in creating summary reports, presentations, abstracts etc.
- Research skills and strong computer skills, Word, PowerPoint, Excel
- Strong interpersonal skills and ability to work well within cross-functional teams.
- Ability to identify key issues and take appropriate actions to address them
- And most importantly: an individual with enthusiasm, energy, drive and initiative

SOCSCI 2EL0

What the student will gain:

- Core understanding of the Canadian healthcare environment and issues facing the pharmaceutical industry
- Understanding the requirements for drug reimbursement in different Canadian jurisdictions.
- Understanding legislation and government policy and how they affect industry and consumers
- Opportunity to develop core pieces of information used by the entire organization
- Freedom to take on projects of interest which will add value to the department, the company and the student
- Involvement in developing market access plans for major products
- The chance to work with a dynamic, rapidly evolving company

As this is an extended work term, the student will be able to participate fully in major product initiatives, develop long-term strategies and tactics and lead major projects

| | |
|---|---|
| **All Degrees and Disciplines** | No |
| **Number of Positions** | 1 |
| **Internship Work Schedule** | Monday - Friday |
| **Hours per Week** | 35-40 |
| **Position Start Date** | May 2016 |
| **Position End Date** | December 2016 |
| **Duration** | 8 months |

## APPLICATION INFORMATION

| | |
|---|---|
| **Application Procedure** | OSCARplus |
| **Application Material Required** | Cover Letter |
| | Resume |

**Additional Application Information**

Please ensure that you are using simple fonts (i.e. Arial, Times) and that you PDF each document before uploading to OSCARplus. Be sure to double check your application package for any formatting errors.

**\*NOTE:** Employers may request students bring a copy of their official transcript to scheduled interviews. Please ensure to obtain copies of your transcript from the Registrar's Office or from the Faculty Office (KTH 129) as early as possible.

**If your application contains errors, omissions, or is of poor quality, it reflects negatively on you as well as the Experiential Education Office and will therefore NOT be passed on to the employer for consideration.**

*Students are not to contact the employer directly under any circumstances!*

SOCSCI 2EL0

## Job Posting: 52543 - Position: Research Intern

| | |
|---|---|
| **Application Deadline** | 06/30/2016 4:00 PM |
| **Application Method:** | OSCARplus |
| **Posting Goes Live:** | 06/18/2016 10:12 AM |
| **Job Posting Status:** | Expired |

## ORGANIZATION INFORMATION

| | |
|---|---|
| **Organization** | Higher Education Quality Council of Ontario (HECQO) |
| **City** | Toronto |
| **Province / State** | Ontario |
| **Country** | Canada |

## JOB POSTING INFORMATION

| | |
|---|---|
| **Position Type** | Full-time Internship |
| **Position Title** | Research Intern |
| **Position Location** | Toronto, ON |
| **Salary** | $19.40 per hour |

**Position Description**

**TO BE ELIGIBLE TO PARTICIPATE IN THE SOCIAL SCIENCES INTERNSHIP PROGRAM, STUDENTS MUST MEET THE FOLLOWING REQUIREMENTS FROM THE TIME OF APPLICATION.**

Students MUST:

- Registered in 18 units or more in the Faculty of Social Sciences in a degree program for the Fall/Winter 2016/2017 session;
- Be in good academic standing with the university (not on academic probation);
- Be in good financial standing with the university (no outstanding financial accounts on the student record);
- Be registered in Level II or above (Please note that official registration for Level II begins only after the student has successfully completed Level I requirements and has commenced coursework for Level II, usually in September of their second year);
- Have completed SOC SCI 2EL0, Career Planning through Experiential Learning. <u>No exemptions will be made</u>; and
- All internship candidates must be authorized to work in Canada. International students must refer to the Government of Canada website http://www.cic.gc.ca/english/study/work-offcampus.asp to ensure eligibility before submitting an application.

**Please Note:** In addition to the eligibility criteria listed above, students must ensure that the internship placement is completed before degree requirements are fulfilled.

***APPLICATIONS WILL BE SCREENED FOR ELIGIBILITY BEFORE BEING PASSED ON TO THE EMPLOYER.***
SOCSCI 2EL0

HEQCO is seeking skilled students to join its small and dynamic research team. We are looking forward to the opportunity to help you enhance and develop knowledge and skills that will be useful for your career success, as well as familiarize you with the current landscape of public policy research in higher education and with Ontario's postsecondary sector.

Reporting to one of HEQCO's executive directors, the research intern may be responsible for any or all of the following: *conducting literature reviews, developing surveys and performing scans on policy development
*writing and preparing requests for proposals, briefings, reports, graphs, tables and presentations for senior researchers
*assisting in the analysis and evaluation of data using software such as STATA or SPSS
*organizing and/or participating in projects, workshops, conferences, etc.

As the research intern, you will be involved in a number of research activities. You will collaborate with senior HEQCO colleagues on research projects where you will be exposed to a variety of research methods in public policy. Your work will normally be guided by a HEQCO researcher who will assist in developing your skills and knowledge and provide guidance and advice during your internship.

**Position Requirements**

- currently enrolled in an undergraduate program
- organized, self-motivated and able to work both independently and as part of a team
- exceptional written and verbal communication skills
- experience in applied research utilizing quantitative and/or qualitative methods
- relevant work, volunteer and/or extracurricular experience
- a demonstrated interest in the postsecondary sector, particularly in Ontario

| | |
|---|---|
| **All Degrees and Disciplines** | Yes |
| **Number of Positions** | 1 |
| **Internship Work Schedule** | Monday - Friday |
| **Hours per Week** | 35-40 |
| **Position Start Date** | September 2016 |
| **Position End Date** | December 2016 |
| **Duration** | 4 months |

## APPLICATION INFORMATION

| | |
|---|---|
| **Application Procedure** | OSCARplus |
| **If by eMail, send to** | hr@heqco.ca |
| **Application Material Required** | Cover Letter |
| | Resume |

SOCSCI 2EL0

**Additional Application Information**

This is a 2-step application process:

1.    Apply through OSCARplus

AND

2.    Apply to: hr@heqco.ca

Please ensure that you are using simple fonts (i.e. Arial, Times) and that you PDF each document before uploading to OSCARplus. Be sure to double check your application package for any formatting errors.

**\*NOTE:**   Employers may request students bring a copy of their official transcript to scheduled interviews. Please ensure to obtain copies of your transcript from the Registrar's Office or from the Faculty Office (KTH 129) as early as possible.

**If your application contains errors, omissions, or is of poor quality, it reflects negatively on you as well as the Experiential Education Office and will therefore NOT be passed on to the employer for consideration.**

*Students are not to contact the employer directly under any circumstances!*

SOCSCI 2EL0

# WEEK 3

SOC SCI 2ELO

45

# SOCSCI 2EL0 COVER LETTER RUBRIC

**\*\*You must receive a minimum of 23/25 as part of the PASS of 2EL0. Each bullet beneath is worth 1 point for a total of 25 points (25 bullets in total). Please refer to the course outline for further details.**

| | STUDENT | INSTRUCTOR: |
|---|---|---|
| **FORMATTING:** | | |
| **Font** | ☐ ☐ ☐ ☐ ☐ | ☐ Easy to read, professional looking font (Tahoma, Arial, Verdana, Times New Roman, etc.)<br>☐ Size: 10.5-12 *point font*<br>☐ Consistent font size and style between resume and cover letter<br>☐ Name no larger than 16 points and bolded<br>☐ No excessive graphics, colour or pictures |
| **Formatting** | ☐ ☐ ☐ ☐ ☐ ☐ | ☐ NO spelling, grammar, or punctuation errors<br>☐ *Single spacing within each paragraph*<br>☐ Cover letter is left justified, no indentations<br>☐ No more than ten "I"s are used throughout<br>☐ Avoids word repetition (i.e. does not use the same verbs to start sentences or to describe various accomplishments)<br>☐ Did not copy language from courseware example |
| **Name, Address, Coordinates** | ☐ ☐ | ☐ Personal information is located at the top of the letter and matches resume header format<br>☐ Addressed to a specific name where possible, or *Hiring Manager or Recruitment Team* |
| **CONTENT:** | | |
| **Introduction (1st Paragraph)** | ☐ ☐ ☐ | ☐ Powerful and unique opening sentence - the first paragraph should be the strongest<br>☐ Includes the company name and job title<br>☐ Identifies how the student heard about the position (online, OSCARplus etc.) |
| **Achievement Oriented (2nd Paragraph) \*2 columns is okay** | ☐ ☐ ☐ ☐ ☐ | ☐ Top three **applicable** skills directly related to job description are clearly identified in first sentence<br>☐ First skill follows SAR formula (Situation Action Result) as per week 2 in courseware<br>☐ Second skill follows SAR formula (Situation Action Result) as per week 2 in courseware<br>☐ Third skill follows SAR formula (Situation Action Result) as per week 2 in courseware<br>☐ No passive statements (e.g. "I was responsible for..." as this does not show how or why) |
| **Research/why you are interested (3rd Paragraph)** | ☐ ☐ ☐ | ☐ Knowledge of the company is demonstrated and connected to personal interests/values<br>☐ Information is not repeated from the company's website, rather paraphrased<br>☐ The focus is on what student can do for the company <u>not</u> what the company can do for the student |
| **Closing paragraph (4th Paragraph)** | ☐ | ☐ Thanks the employer for consideration |

**NOTES: To be filled by Instructor**

**INSTRUCTOR SCORE:**

## /25

**\*must achieve a minimum of 23/25**

# MY JOB MATCH CHART

Using ONE of the supplied job postings included in your courseware, answer the following questions based on the information provided in the posting. **Once complete upload to your PebblePad portfolio**.

**Position**

| Job Title | |
|-----------|---|
| Employer | |

Be sure to focus on your skills, education and other qualifications!

| Employer "Wants" (I possess) | Where did I gain this qualification? |
|------------------------------|--------------------------------------|
| | |
| | |
| | |
| | |
| | |
| | |

| Employer "Wants" (I need to develop) | Where can I gain this qualification? |
|--------------------------------------|--------------------------------------|
| | |
| | |
| | |
| | |

SOC SCI 2EL0

# COVER LETTER IN-CLASS ACTIVITY

1. Using the job description chosen from your courseware, practice formatting a cover letter based on the first four cover letter writing components as per the class PowerPoint:

## 2. Your opening paragraph:

_____

_____

_____

_____

## 3. SAR Activity:

| Situation | Action | Result |
|-----------|--------|--------|
|           |        |        |

Accomplishment Statement:

_____

_____

_____

_____

# YOUR GUIDE TO COVER LETTER WRITING

## First Paragraph – *What You Want*

- Introduce yourself with a powerful opening
- Capture reader's interest indicating 2-3 key strengths that align with the role
- Include brief details about how you heard of the opening
- Keep this paragraph strong but brief; one sentence preferred

**Before:** *I am writing in response to your posting on OSCARplus for a Research Assistant position.*

**After:** *With three years of part-time work experience managing case reviews and honing qualitative and quantitative research methods through my academic career, I have developed the skills necessary to excel in the Research Assistant role for ABC Company, as posted on the OSCARplus website at McMaster University.*

## Second Paragraph – *How You Fit*

- This can be done in traditional or two column format
- Highlight three things (skills, knowledge, experience) that align closely with the role or company requirements; these need to align with the job description
- Use SAR to briefly explain how you demonstrated each skill, to create interest around your accomplishments (results); what you did, how you did it, what the outcome was
- If appropriate, identify gaps and describe how you would close these gaps for employer (i.e. – if a company required experience with a software application that you are not familiar with, explain how you have quickly learned new applications in the past)

**Before:** *My experience and training in management techniques is enhanced by my strong work ethic and ability to learn new concepts quickly. I am an excellent communicator, a results-oriented performer and get great satisfaction from making a difference. I thoroughly enjoy working with people and have done so throughout my career. I bring top results in managing a retail operation.*

**After:** *Through my extracurricular and work experiences, I have demonstrated strong leadership, communication and problem solving skills. As the Co-Chair of the Social Sciences Program Fair, I managed a group of six committee members, by empowering and assessing individual strengths to delegate tasks and organize a successful one-day event for over 200 first and second year students. In addition, I have refined my communication skills as a Sales Associate at Best Buy. By actively listening and adjusting my sales pitch to potential customers to promote specific product attributes, I achieved daily sales targets of $2K while consistently providing excellent customer service. Finally, in a third year research methods course, I partnered with four other team members to effectively analyze programs offered within a Hamilton based social services organization. Through the utilization of qualitative, quantitative, and statistical analysis, our team identified problems within the program delivery and areas for improvement, which were provided in summary of recommendations to the organization. One of the proposals was later implemented by the association, increasing community engagement opportunities by five percent in 2016.*

SOC SCI 2EL0

### Third Paragraph – *Why You Are Interested*

- Explain why you are interested in the position – it tells the employer how motivated you are for the role
- Do research and include information that demonstrates your knowledge of the company or industry (i.e. you are impressed by the innovative green initiatives – DO NOT repeat sections of company website)
- Do not include ambiguous or vague sentences that cannot be directly tied back to your skills, experience, or knowledge (i.e. I am able to quickly adapt to changing situations and requirements)
- Be careful not to focus on what the company can do for you, but what you can do for the company

**Before:** *I have always wanted to work at ABC Company, and I would be very interested to conduct research and provide excellent customer service for your department.*

**After:** *ABC Company is renowned for customer service and community involvement. My previous experience at Best Buy has taught me that a commitment to customer service is required whenever new policies, practices and processes are implemented. I am confident that my experience will contribute to your organization as it continues to strive for customer service excellence in existing and new markets.*

### Fourth Paragraph – *Closing and Follow-up*

- Let the employer know when you will follow up (not for internship recruitment as EE will do this on your behalf)
- Be confident in your closing – you are not done marketing yourself until you have signed the letter
- Leave the employer with a positive impression of what you have to offer
- Thank the employer for their consideration; do not reiterate contact information

**Before:** *I hope that you will review my resume and will consider me for the position. I would love to work at your company more than anything. Please contact me at xxx-xxx-xxxx or email me at xxx@mcmaster.ca anytime.*

**After:** *I am eager to help advance the success of the Research Department at ABC Company and I look forward to the opportunity to discuss my suitability for this role with you further. Thank you for your consideration.*

# John Doe
123 Main Street West, Hamilton, Ontario L8P 1H9
(905) 123-4567 | doej@mcmaster.ca
www.linkedin.com/in/johndoe

November 8, 2017

Ron Neumann
Executive Director
Innovation Factory
175 Longwood Road South
Hamilton, Ontario L8P 0A1

RE: Business Development Coordinator

Dear Mr. Neumann,

Three years of diverse work experience demanding that I swiftly grasp the nature of the business and deliver results under minimal supervision makes me an excellent candidate for the position of Business Development Coordinator at Innovation Factory as posted on McMaster University's job board.

Through these experiences I have developed strong analytical, leadership, and customer service skills. I enhanced my analytical skills through my role as an Executive Board member for the McMaster Students Union where my duty was to advise the Board of Directors on how policy decisions would affect day-to-day operations of the organization. As a Camp Counsellor, strong leadership was essential when supervising 11 children while facilitating daily activities focused on basketball skill development and team building. While employed at the Canada Border Services Agency last summer as an Administrative and Communications Support Intern, my customer service skills were utilized when I developed a comprehensive communications strategy to ensure cohesive messages were delivered to upwards of 5,000 internal and external stakeholders.

While reading the recent article about your organization featured in the October issue of the Hamilton Business Magazine, I was impressed to learn of your involvement in community and business fundraising activities for local organizations. With eight years of volunteer activities in non-profit organizations, I look forward to joining such a reputable community centred company.

A meeting to discuss my experience and skills as they relate to your current or future needs would be appreciated. Please feel free to contact me in the meantime with any questions or to arrange an interview. Thank you for your time and consideration.

Sincerely,

*John Doe*

John Doe

Encl.: Resume -2 pages

SOC SCI 2EL0

# John Doe
123 Main Street West, Hamilton, Ontario L8P 1H9
(905) 123-4567 | doej@mcmaster.ca
www.linkedin.com/in/johndoe

November 8, 2017

Ron Neumann
Executive Director
Innovation Factory
175 Longwood Road South
Hamilton, Ontario L8P 0A1

Re: Business Development Coordinator

Dear Mr. Neumann,

Three years of diverse work experience demanding that I swiftly grasp the nature of the business and deliver results under minimal supervision makes me an excellent candidate for the position of Business Development Coordinator at Innovation Factory as posted on McMaster University's job board.

**Customer Service**

Developed a comprehensive communications strategy for the Canada Border Services Agency to ensure cohesive messages were delivered to upwards of 5,000 stakeholders.

**Leadership**

As a Camp Counselor, supervised 11 children while facilitating daily activities focused on basketball skill development and team building.

**Analytical Skills**

Served a term as an Executive Board member for the McMaster Students Union. Advised the Board of Directors on how policy decisions would affect day-to-day operations of the organization.

While reading the recent article about your organization featured in the October issue of the Hamilton Business Magazine, I was impressed to learn of your involvement in community and business fundraising activities for local organizations. With eight years of volunteer activities in non-profit organizations, I look forward to joining such a reputable community centred company.

A meeting to discuss my experience and skills as they relate to your current or future needs would be appreciated. Please feel free to contact me in the meantime with any questions or to arrange an interview. Thank you for your time and consideration.

Sincerely,

*John Doe*

John Doe

encl.: Resume - 2 pages

SOC SCI 2EL0

# WEEK 4

SOC SCI 2ELO

# SOCSCI 2EL0 RESUME RUBRIC

**\*\*You must receive a minimum of 27/30 as part of the PASS of 2EL0. Each bullet beneath is worth 1 point for a total of 30 points (30 bullets in total). Please refer to the course outline for further details.**

| | STUDENT | INSTRUCTOR | FORMATTING: |
|---|---|---|---|
| **Font** | ☐ | ☐ | Easy to read, professional looking font (Tahoma, Arial, Verdana, Times New Roman, etc.) |
| | ☐ | ☐ | Size: 10.5-12 point font |
| | ☐ | ☐ | Consistent font size and style between resume and cover letter |
| | ☐ | ☐ | Name no larger than 16 points and bolded |
| | ☐ | ☐ | No excessive graphics, colour or pictures |
| **Formatting** | ☐ | ☐ | Single spacing within each section |
| | ☐ | ☐ | Headers are discernible at a glance and consistent throughout – can be 13-14 point font |
| | ☐ | ☐ | Well-balanced margins and no under/over use of white space |
| | ☐ | ☐ | Dates aligned on the right |
| | ☐ | ☐ | Months written out in full |
| | ☐ | ☐ | NO "Objective" or "Skills" section |
| | ☐ | ☐ | Use of bullets, no paragraphs |
| | ☐ | ☐ | Reverse chronological order |
| **Your Contact Info** | ☐ | ☐ | Personal information is located at the top of the letter and matches cover letter header format |

| | STUDENT | INSTRUCTOR | CONTENT: |
|---|---|---|---|
| | ☐ | ☐ | NO spelling, grammar or punctuation errors |
| | ☐ | ☐ | Numbers 1-10 are written in full, 11+ in numerical format |
| | ☐ | ☐ | Correct use of abbreviations written in full first, followed by abbreviation in brackets |
| | ☐ | ☐ | Bullets do not start with or include "Responsible for" |
| | ☐ | ☐ | No first person references: "I" or "My" |
| **HIGHLIGHTS** | ☐ | ☐ | Maximum 6 bullets |
| | ☐ | ☐ | Tailored to the job – just by reading this section, the reader knows the type of job you are applying to |
| **EDUCATION** | ☐ | ☐ | Degree on 1st line and bolded |
| | ☐ | ☐ | Academic Institution on line two |
| | ☐ | ☐ | Courses are relevant to specific job and defined, not just listed |
| **EXPERIENCE** | ☐ | ☐ | Paid and unpaid experience are listed with the same format |
| | ☐ | ☐ | Job title is the only item bolded |
| | ☐ | ☐ | Use of the SAR format for each bullet: (as per week 3 in courseware) **S** – what **skill** is being demonstrated **A** – what **action** did you take **R** – what was the **result** of your action |
| | ☐ | ☐ | Uses different action verbs at the beginning of each bullet throughout resume – no repetition |
| | ☐ | ☐ | Bullets start with past tense action verbs |
| **INTERESTS** | ☐ | ☐ | Are not just listed, rather includes specific details of involvement, frequency, etc... |

| NOTES: To be filled by Instructor |
|---|

| INSTRUCTOR SCORE: **/30** *must achieve a minimum of 27/30 | |
|---|---|

# YOUR GUIDE TO RESUME WRITING

**What is a resume?**

Resumes are what people use to get jobs, right?

Wrong!

A resume is a one or two page summary of your education, skills, accomplishments and experience. Your resume's purpose is to get your foot in the door. A resume does its job successfully if it does not exclude you from consideration. Your resume is your ticket to an interview where you can sell yourself!

**How to Prepare an Effective Resume**

*1. The Essentials*

Before you write, take time to do a self-assessment on paper. Outline your skills and abilities as well as your work experience and extracurricular activities. This will make it easier to prepare a thorough resume.

*2. The Content Of Your Resume*

| PRESENTATION | |
|---|---|
| ☐ | Font<br>• Use a simple, easy to read font with a maximum of two font types (one for headers, one for body)<br>• 10.5 – 12 point font (name should be no larger than 16 point font) (headers can be 13-14 point font) |
| ☐ | Format<br>• Use the same heading format on your resume and cover letter<br>• Ensure resume sections are clearly defined and bolded or underlined, and in order of importance and relevance<br>• Use single spacing within each section; margins should be no less than 0.5" and no greater than 1" and even on both sides, top and bottom<br>• Dates, titles and employers are discernible at a glance and consistent formatting is used<br>• Dates should be included in full at right margin (i.e. January – October 2016). Months may not be necessary<br>• Use white paper<br>• When emailing application, convert to pdf format<br>• Print on one side of the paper<br>• Resume is between 1.5 – 2 pages in length<br>• Ensure name and page number are at the top of the second page<br>• White space is used well, resume is visually appealing<br>• Language settings on Word – English Canadian if applying to Canadian jobs<br>• Be mindful using a template – this is YOUR marketing paper, not a template |

SOC SCI 2EL0

| | |
|---|---|
| ☐ | **First Impressions**<br>• First page of resume should include the strongest content<br>• *An employer takes less than a minute to determine if they want to read any further*- ensure that you have the relevant information that will capture their interest |
| **ORDER OF CONTENT** | |
| ☐ | **Contact information**<br>• Name (in larger font than body of resume), home address, phone number (with area code) & email are at the top of resume<br>• Email is appropriate and not hyperlinked<br>• Avoid nicknames<br>• Be mindful of the phone number you include (if you have an answering service, record a neutral greeting)<br>• Include your LinkedIn url – make sure you customize it |
| ☐ | **Objective or Summary**<br>• To use only if you are NOT including a cover letter<br>• An objective tells potential employers the work you're hoping to do.<br>• Be specific about the job you want<br>• Tailor your objective to each employer you target/every job you are seeking |
| ☐ | **Highlights of Qualifications**<br>• 3 – 5 bullets<br>• Specific to each job – a generic highlights section does NOT work<br>• Should be able to distinguish the type of role applying to just from reading this section |
| ☐ | **Education**<br>• List your education in reverse chronological order - that is, put your most recent education first and work backward<br>• Include degree, major/specialization on first line in bold; university name, location and date on second line not in bold (italics preferred)<br>• Add your grade point average (GPA) if it is higher than 8 or 9<br>• Define relevant courses, projects completed<br>• Include internships, and other academic activities completed<br>• Mention academic honours/awards |
| ☐ | **Paid and Unpaid Experience**<br>• List your experience in reverse chronological order - that is, put your most recent experience first and work backward<br>• Format all experience the same and ensure you provide the following:<br><br>**Title of position (bold)**                              Dates of employment<br>Name of organization, City, Province<br>• Need bullets showcasing accomplishments, not a listing of duties<br>• Apply "Bullet Points" and "Action Verbs" list on next page |

**SOC SCI 2EL0**

62

|   | Bullet points |
|---|---|
|   | • Use bullet points- 3-5 per relevant experience |
|   | • *One sentence only per bullet point*; use semicolons sparingly to connect similar/related ideas into one bullet |
|   | • Most significant and/or relevant aspects of the role should be in first bullet, followed by bullets in descending order of importance |
|   | • Ensure consistent use of periods throughout resume (all or none) |
|   | **Action Verbs** |
|   | • Use past tense even if currently in the role |
|   | • Use different descriptors and verbs throughout and try to limit word/phrase repetition *Refer to Action Verbs* handout |
| ☐ | **Make it Unique** |
|   | • Use additional sections such as Volunteer Experience, Extra-Curricular Activities and Interests to demonstrate your well-roundedness as a candidate by promoting your extracurricular involvement |
|   | • Do not underestimate the value of any experience (i.e. summer employment, family business) |
|   | • Be specific when including interests (i.e. Music- do you play an instrument?) and include activities that include your uniqueness (i.e. photography, art, sports etc…) |
|   | • If Interests are included, they have been selected mindfully to add value and highlight relevant skills and not just listed, rather defined |
| ☐ | **References:** |
|   | • Ask people if they are willing to serve as references **before** you give their names to a potential employer. |
|   | • Do not include your reference information on your resume. You may note at the bottom of your resume: "References available upon request." |
| | **CONTENT** |
| ☐ | **Achievement Orientation** |
|   | • Make use of SAR statements to demonstrate what, why, how, when and the result |
|   | • Relevant experience must include results/outcomes and quantify where possible |
|   | • Do not simply list your duties or tasks |
|   | • Skills and accomplishments are emphasized, rather than duties or responsibilities (i.e. "balanced budget 99% of time", NOT "responsible for budget") |
|   | • Skills are qualified and accomplishments are quantified where possible |
|   | • Do not use "Responsible for", it can come off as weak and passive |
|   | • Remain objective, do not use "I" or "Me" pronouns |
| ☐ | **Concise and Varied** |
|   | • Reduce your word count where possible (i.e. "to" vs. "in order to") |
|   | • Prune your words and avoid repetition (same verbs to describe all accomplishments |

**SOC SCI 2EL0**

| | |
|---|---|
| ☐ | **Error-Free**<br>• Ensure no spelling or grammatical mistakes<br>• Ask *many people to proofread. The more people who see your resume, the* more likely that misspelled words and awkward phrases will be noticed |
| ☐ | **Using Numbers**<br>• Spell out numbers from one to ten; use number format for 11 and above<br>• Avoid adding the word "dollar" after $200 (symbol identifies this as a dollar amount)<br>• To maximize space use $100K instead of $100,000 |
| ☐ | **Abbreviations/Acronyms**<br>• Spell out months and university degrees in full (Bachelor of Arts vs. BA)<br>• Avoid using abbreviations, except for Provinces and States (ON, AB, NY)<br>• If using acronyms, spell out completely the first time, followed by acronym in brackets; acronyms can be used for the rest of the document |

**SOC SCI 2EL0**

# ACTION VERBS

## Communication/People Skills

- Addressed
- Advertised
- Arbitrated
- Arranged
- Articulated
- Authored
- Clarified
- Collaborated
- Communicated
- Composed
- Condensed
- Conferred
- Consulted
- Contacted
- Conveyed
- Convinced
- Corresponded
- Debated
- Defined
- Developed
- Directed
- Discussed
- Drafted
- Edited
- Elicited
- Enlisted
- Explained
- Expressed
- Formulated
- Furnished
- Incorporated
- Influenced
- Interacted
- Interpreted
- Interviewed
- Involved
- Joined
- Judged
- Lectured
- Listened
- Marketed
- Mediated
- Moderated
- Negotiated
- Observed
- Outlined
- Participated
- Persuaded
- Presented
- Promoted
- Proposed
- Publicized
- Reconciled
- Recruited
- Referred
- Reinforced
- Reported
- Resolved
- Responded
- Solicited
- Specified
- Spoke
- Suggested
- Summarized
- Synthesized
- Translated
- Wrote

## Creative Skills

- Acted
- Adapted
- Began
- Combined
- Composed
- Conceptualized
- Condensed
- Created
- Customized
- Designed
- Developed
- Directed
- Displayed
- Drew
- Entertained
- Established
- Fashioned
- Formulated
- Founded
- Illustrated
- Initiated
- Instituted
- Integrated
- Introduced
- Invented
- Modeled
- Modified
- Originated
- Performed
- Photographed
- Planned
- Revised
- Revitalized
- Shaped
- Solved

## Data/Financial Skills

- Administered
- Adjusted
- Allocated
- Analyzed
- Appraised
- Assessed
- Audited
- Balanced
- Budgeted
- Calculated
- Computed
- Conserved
- Corrected
- Determined
- Developed
- Estimated
- Forecasted
- Managed
- Marketed
- Measured
- Netted
- Planned
- Prepared
- Programmed
- Projected
- Qualified
- Reconciled
- Reduced
- Researched
- Retrieved

Source: http://www.quintcareers.com

## Helping Skills

- Adapted
- Advocated
- Aided
- Answered
- Arranged
- Assessed
- Assisted
- Clarified
- Coached
- Collaborated
- Contributed
- Cooperated
- Counseled
- Demonstrated
- Diagnosed
- Educated
- Encouraged
- Ensured
- Expedited
- Facilitated
- Familiarized
- Furthered
- Guided
- Helped
- Insured
- Intervened
- Motivated
- Prevented
- Provided
- Referred
- Rehabilitated
- Represented
- Resolved
- Simplified
- Supplied
- Supported
- Volunteered

## Management/Leadership Skills

- Administered
- Analyzed
- Appointed
- Approved
- Assigned
- Attained
- Authorized
- Chaired
- Considered
- Consolidated
- Contracted
- Controlled
- Converted
- Coordinated
- Decided
- Delegated
- Developed
- Directed
- Eliminated
- Emphasized
- Enforced
- Enhanced
- Established
- Executed
- Generated
- Handled
- Headed
- Hired
- Hosted
- Improved
- Incorporated
- Increased
- Initiated
- Inspected
- Instituted
- Led
- Managed
- Merged
- Motivated
- Navigated
- Organized
- Originated
- Overhauled
- Oversaw
- Planned
- Presided
- Prioritized
- Produced
- Recommended
- Reorganized
- Replaced
- Restored
- Reviewed
- Scheduled
- Secured
- Selected
- Streamlined
- Strengthened
- Supervised
- Terminated

## Organizational Skills

- Approved
- Arranged
- Catalogued
- Categorized
- Charted
- Classified
- Coded
- Collected
- Compiled
- Corrected
- Corresponded
- Distributed
- Executed
- Filed
- Generated
- Incorporated
- Inspected
- Logged
- Maintained
- Monitored
- Obtained
- Operated
- Ordered
- Organized
- Prepared
- Processed
- Provided
- Purchased
- Recorded
- Registered
- Reserved
- Responded
- Reviewed
- Routed
- Scheduled
- Screened
- Submitted
- Supplied
- Standardized
- Systematized
- Updated
- Validated
- Verified

Source: http://www.quintcareers.com

## Research Skills

- Analyzed
- Clarified
- Collected
- Compared
- Conducted
- Critiqued
- Detected
- Determined
- Diagnosed
- Evaluated
- Examined
- Experimented
- Explored
- Extracted
- Formulated
- Gathered
- Inspected
- Interviewed
- Invented
- Investigated
- Located
- Measured
- Organized
- Researched
- Reviewed
- Searched
- Solved
- Summarized
- Surveyed
- Systematized
- Tested

## Teaching Skills

- Adapted
- Advised
- Clarified
- Coached
- Communicated
- Conducted
- Coordinated
- Critiqued
- Developed
- Enabled
- Encouraged
- Evaluated
- Explained
- Facilitated
- Focused
- Guided
- Individualized
- Informed
- Instilled
- Instructed
- Motivated
- Persuaded
- Simulated
- Stimulated
- Taught
- Tested
- Trained
- Transmitted
- Tutored

## Technical Skills

- Adapted
- Applied
- Assembled
- Built
- Calculated
- Computed
- Conserved
- Constructed
- Converted
- Debugged
- Designed
- Determined
- Developed
- Engineered
- Fabricated
- Fortified
- Installed
- Maintained
- Operated
- Overhauled
- Printed
- Programmed
- Rectified
- Regulated
- Remodeled
- Repaired
- Replaced
- Restored
- Solved
- Specialized
- Standardized
- Studied
- Upgraded
- Utilized

Source: http://www.quintcareers.com

# ACCOMPLISHMENT STATEMENTS

The best way to tailor your resume is to write accomplishment statements for every bullet point that clearly demonstrates what you did vs. simply listing duties or responsibilities

Accomplishment statements show how you can add value to an employer's team or organization based on what you've done in the past.

Always begin with a strong action verb.

## Skill + Action + Result = Accomplishment Statement

### Accomplishment Statement Examples:

**Before**: Started a new program
**After**: Created and implemented a new mentoring program with 80% participation of residents

**Before**: Helped in research study
**After**: Contributed to an analytical research study using Quasi-experimental methods and experimental designs, creating detailed reports

**Before**: Stocked shelves
**After**: Maintained merchandise supply to ensure availability of products to customers by using XYZ's computerized inventory system

**Before**: Answered calls from angry customers
**After**: Responded to approximately 25 calls per day from dissatisfied customers; successfully answered inquiries and satisfied their concerns, resulting in de-escalation of claims

**Before**: Responsible for obtaining new members
**After**: Increased membership in ABC student club by 50% through creative social media advertising

**Before**: Took food orders and served hamburgers and fries
**After**: Responded to customers in a timely and effective manner in a fast paced environment, ensuring accurate orders

**SOC SCI 2EL0**

# SAR Activity (In class exercise)

| Skill | Action | Result |
|-------|--------|--------|
|       |        |        |

Accomplishment Statement:

_____

_____

_____

_____

| Skill | Action | Result |
|-------|--------|--------|
|       |        |        |

Accomplishment Statement:

_____

_____

_____

_____

**SOC SCI 2EL0**

# NAME

Street Name
City, Province Postal Code

(905) 123-4567
appropriate.email@gmail.com

## KEY ACHIEVEMENTS:

- Quantify your relevant experience if possible (e.g. Over two years' experience working in....)
- Academic work that relates to the job you are applying for (e.g. Completed written research report and presentation on sociological impacts related to deviant youth and alcohol abuse)
- Skills developed through volunteer placement(s) that relates to the job you are applying for (e.g. Created functional databases and kept confidential and accurate up-to-date records for ABC Volunteer Agency)
- Award or Recognition Received (e.g. Received the Dr. Mary E. Keyes Certificate of Leadership for completion of workshops and community service, McMaster University, April 2016)

## EDUCATION:

**Completing Bachelor of Arts (Sociology)**                               2014 – present
McMaster University, Hamilton ON

- Expected graduation date: April 2018
- Relevant Projects: describe completed projects relevant to position
- List awards received and for what (e.g. Invited to join the Golden Key Honour Society for Academic Excellence) etc.
- Internship Positions (e.g. Completed an internship placement with the Canadian Space Agency as a Research Assistant (September 2015 – April 2016)
- Membership/positions in student run academic clubs (e.g. Member of the Pre-Law Society)
- Relevant Courses: course names and descriptions relevant to position (do not list course codes)

## EXPERIENCE:

**Research Assistant** – Internship Position                               Date
Canadian Space Agency

- Outline major accomplishments of position (e.g. Performed literature searches and reviews regarding information related to human physical reactions to the space environment)
- State any unique achievements (e.g. Presented research findings at Departmental meetings and outlined recommendations for changes to current programming which will be implemented in 2018)
- Mention major achievements/recognitions (e.g. Recognized by supervising staff members for excellent team-work and superior written communication skills exhibited throughout the placement)
- List any computer/new technology used (e.g. Utilized software including SPSS, Microsoft Excel and Access database programs for compiling and analyzing statistical information)

## EXPERIENCE CONTINUED...

**Summer Camp Program Coordinator** – Volunteer                    Date
ABC Volunteer Agency
- Summarize accomplishments using numbers where possible (e.g. Worked closely with social workers, parents and camps to create and implement a streamlined registration process for over 200 children ages 6-12)
- Outline major tasks of the position (e.g. Matched client behaviour profiles with suitable programs and performed safety evaluations for each camp, providing recommendations for improvement to the program)
- Summarize administrative accomplishments last (e.g. Arranged for transportation of campers, and completed data entry to ensure accurate and up to date records)

**Customer Service Associate** - Part-Time Position                    Date
Wal-Mart Canada Inc.
- Use monetary values to show responsibility (e.g. Managed and balanced a cash float of approximately $500 daily)
- Outline your customer service skills (e.g. Handled customer requests and concerns effectively and notified management when necessary)
- Mention any recognitions (e.g. Recognized as "Associate of the Month" for outstanding customer service five times over a two year period)
- List committee affiliations (e.g. Member of the Health and Safety Committee - worked as part of a team or four to ensure a safe work environment for all employees)

## AWARDS AND RECOGNITIONS

**Dr. Mary E. Keyes Certificate of Leadership**                    Date
- State reason for recognition (e.g. Completed leadership workshops at McMaster University, including....)

**Student Experience Grant Recipient**                    Date
- State reason for award (e.g. Received $500 grant used to travel to Africa to volunteer in an orphanage providing health care to children)

## EXTRA CURRICULAR ACTIVITIES

**President of the McMaster Photography Club**                    Date
- Outline major accomplishments (e.g. Organized three general meetings and two events per year, raising membership by 20%)

**MacServe Participant**                    Date
- Outline event and what you accomplished (e.g. Participated in a half-day volunteer event with a team of 11 volunteers painting a room at the Good Shepherd Centre)

**Job Shadow Week Participant**                    Date
- Outline event and what you accomplished (e.g. Participated in a half-day job shadow experience with an Addictions Counsellor to learn more about the field)

## REFERENCES AVAILABLE UPON REQUEST

SOC SCI 2EL0

# JOHN DOE

123 Main Street West, Hamilton, Ontario L8P 1H9
(905) 123-4567 | doej@mcmaster.ca
www.linkedin.com/in/johndoe

## SUMMARY OF QUALIFICATIONS

- Experience in research, including analyzing data and performing statistical formulations.
- Presented Economic research findings at a conference in New York City.
- Refined public speaking skills through participation in Toastmasters.
- Knowledge of the French language with intermediate competency in written and oral communication.
- Proficient in all Microsoft Office Suite, including: Word, Excel, Outlook, PowerPoint and Access.

## EDUCATION

**Candidate for Bachelor of Arts, Honours Economics & Political Science**
*McMaster University, Hamilton, ON*                     September 2014 - Present
- Admitted to Golden Key Honour Society for Academic Excellence.
- Completed a full time summer internship with *Canada Border Services Agency*.
- Awarded a Student Experience Grant to present at the Economics and Society conference in New York City in January 2016. Research paper topic: *"Forecasting Structure and Time Varying Patterns in Economics and Finance."*
- Expected to graduate in June 2018.
- Relevant Courses:
    - Monetary Economics: Analyzed monetary theory and policy, including money demand and supply, money and inflation and asset market analysis.
    - Financial Economics: Detailed investigation of the financial sector (bond markets, stock markets, financial statements and taxation).

## RELEVANT EXPERIENCE

**Executive Board Member**
*McMaster Students Union, Hamilton, ON*                     May 2017 - Present
- Formulated management and strategic planning decisions on behalf of organization regarding volunteers, staff, services, finances and operations.
- Approved $7M dollar annual operating budget, large expenditure requests and the reallocation of funds within budget categories.
- Advised Board of Directors on how policy decisions affect day-to-day operations of the organization.
- Enhanced understanding and knowledge of the operations, governance and organizational structure of non-profit organizations

SOC SCI 2EL0

**Administrative and Communications Support Intern**
*Canada Border Services Agency, Hamilton, ON*                    May - August 2017
- Created organizational policy manuals to effectively communicate internal strategies and optimize the operations of the department.
- Developed a comprehensive communications strategy and managed all social media outlets to ensure cohesive messages were delivered to upwards of 5,000 internal and external stakeholders.
- Prepared databases and performed merges for large mail-outs using Excel, ensuring timely distribution to external clients.
- Handled reception of visitors, transfer of calls and general inquiries, delivering quality customer service and upholding the government profile.

**Shift Supervisor**
*Starbucks Coffee, Hamilton, ON*                    September 2014 - April 2017
- Delegated tasks such as brewing coffee, cashier, cleaning front or barrister based on personal strengths and interests to a team of six shift employees, which motivated them to perform tasks to best of ability.
- Received Moves of Uncommon Greatness award for receiving 99% store 'Snapshot' based on excellent service provided to secret shopper.
- Coached 16 new employees, one-on-one and delegated responsibility with respect, resulting in increased speed and service to patrons.

**Welcome Week Representative**
*McMaster Social Sciences Society, Hamilton, ON*                    September 2015
- Facilitated events and programs for over 1000 first-year students to help them effectively transition to life at McMaster University.
- Received Welcome Week Cup as a member of faculty team with highest event scores and fundraising total.
- Directed traffic and unloaded belongings for second largest residence during campus move-in day, ensuring the safety of students.

## INTERESTS
- Basketball - Point guard for intramural team at McMaster University.
- Travel - Backpacked across Germany and Switzerland during summer of 2016.
- Golf – Played recreationally for the past ten years.

SOC SCI 2EL0

# WEEK 5

# The Purpose of an Interview

The interview is a mutual exchange of information between an employer and a candidate for a position. The primary objectives are to:

- Supply information about yourself that is not contained in your resume

- Show that you understand yourself and have a sense of direction in your career

- Enable the employer to evaluate your personality and attitudes in terms of the demands of the organization and the position

- Allow you to gain information about the organization and the job, which is not available through other sources

- Give you and the employer an opportunity to discuss the desirability of further contact or an offer of employment

## Preparing for the Interview: Know Yourself

To impress an employer you must be well prepared and understand the value of what you have to offer. To relate your assets to the position and the organization, you must know yourself. Review your self-assessments and your resume. Be prepared to substantiate all points with information. Rather than trying to determine only at what level you are currently functioning, some interviewers want to see how you have grown over time in areas related to their position(s) (e.g., interpersonal and work skills, motivation). Some interviewers will want you to talk about your mistakes to find out what you have learned to do differently.

## Know the Company / Organization

You **must** be familiar with the **position** and the **organization** so that you can demonstrate how and why you will be an effective worker. Refer to the notes you made as you networked with people and reviewed print and online materials.

Obtain information, if you can, on whom you will be meeting with and the schedule for the interview period. If you can find out about your interviewer(s) (e.g., name, title, background) in advance, you will be able to use this information during the interviews.

## The Core of the Interview Process

Don't worry about being nervous during the interview - this is normal and will be expected. Just remember, the interviewer wants to hire you if you have the right qualifications and interest in the position. Many interviewers will begin the interview with some "small talk" to help you relax. This may seem irrelevant to the position, but you are still being evaluated. Take these opening moments to show a positive attitude.

**Used with permission from Career Services, University of Waterloo / Source: Career Development eManual www.cdm.uwaterloo.ca**

The next phase of the interview consists of the interviewer asking you questions to try to determine your fit. Having knowledge of possible questions the employer may ask enables you to prepare points to include in your answers. Think about why the question is being asked. What does the employer really want to know? The following are typical questions an employer may ask:

- Tell me about yourself
- What are your short-term goals? What about in 2 and 5 years from now?
- What is your own vision/mission statement?
- What do you think you will be looking for in the job following this position?
- Why do you feel you will be successful in this work?
- What other types of work are you looking for in addition to this role?
- What supervisory or leadership roles have you had?
- What experience have you had working on a team?
- What have been your most satisfying/disappointing experiences?
- What are your strengths/weaknesses?
- What kinds of problems do you handle the best?
- How do you reduce stress and try to achieve balance in your life?
- How did you handle a request to do something contrary to your moral code or business ethics?
- What was the result the last time you tried to sell your idea to others?
- Why did you apply to our organization and what do you know about us?
- What do you think are advantages/disadvantages of joining our organization?
- What is the most important thing you are looking for in an employer?
- What were some of the common characteristics of your past supervisors?
- What characteristics do you think a person would need to have to work effectively in our company with its policies of staying ahead of the competition?
- What courses did you like best/least? Why?
- What did you learn or gain from your part-time/summer/co-op/internship experiences?
- What are your plans for further studies?
- Why are your grades low?
- How do you spend your spare time?
- If I asked your friends to describe you, what do you think they would say?

- What frustrates you the most?

- When were you last angry at work and what was the outcome?

- What things could you do to increase your overall effectiveness?

- What was the toughest decision you had to make in the last year? Why was it difficult?

- Why haven't you found a job yet?

- You don't seem to have any experience in ___ (e.g., sales, fundraising, bookkeeping), do you?

- Why should I hire you?

## Answering Problem Solving Questions

The interviewer may present a real-life problem or hypothetical situation for you to try and solve. The rationale is that it allows the interviewer to see how a person thinks - how they problem solve. For example:

- A construction engineer might be asked: "What would you do if your crew was digging underground and ran into a rock?"

- A marketer might be asked to come up with 3 strategies to promote a product

- A manager might be asked how they would set up a new manufacturing plant

The key is not to worry about getting the "right" answer, rather, to demonstrate the right way to come up with an answer. Typically, the following 5-step process is appropriate for handling problem solving questions:

1. Listen intently to what is being asked.

2. Ask clarifying questions to determine exactly what the interviewer is looking for.

3. Respond by first explaining how you'd gather the data necessary to make an informed decision.

4. Discuss how you'd use that data to generate options.

5. Finally, based on the data you've gathered, the available options, and your understanding of the open position, explain how you'd make an appropriate decision or recommendation.

Keep in mind, there is no 'right' answer - only 'your' answer. Interviewers often use these types of questions to determine "fit".

# Answering Behaviour-Based Interviewing Questions

One of the most reliable ways for an interviewer to project how you would perform in the future is to examine the past. Therefore, many employers prepare behaviour-based questions. Behaviour-based interviewers usually develop their questions around the traits and skills they deem necessary for succeeding in a position or organization.

They usually begin with phrases like:

"Tell me about a time when..."

"Describe a time when..."

"Give me an example of your _____ skill."

Some candidates find the format of the question unsettling or they simply can't think of anything. However, those who have done research and preparation will have experiences ready. To answer effectively, use the SAR formula – Situation Action Result. Some common behaviour description interview questions are:

Tell me about a time when you demonstrated your ability to...

- Work effectively under pressure
- Handle a difficult situation with a co-worker
- Be creative in solving a problem
- Completed a project on time
- Persuade team members to do things your way
- Write a report that was well-received
- Anticipate potential problems and develop preventative measures
- Make an important decision with limited facts
- Make an unpopular decision
- Adapt to a difficult situation
- Be tolerant of an opinion that was different from yours
- Deal with your disappointment in your behaviour
- Use your political savvy to push a program through that you really believed in
- Deal with an irate customer
- Delegate a project effectively
- Surmount a major obstacle
- Prioritize the elements of a complicated project

**Used with permission from Career Services, University of Waterloo / Source: Career Development eManual www.cdm.uwaterloo.ca**

By analyzing the questions asked of you, you will be able to find out more particulars about the job for which you have applied. What emphasis does the interviewer seem to be placing on which skills, knowledge, personality traits and attitudes? That insight can help you tailor your answers more easily to the employer's position.

## Selling Your Benefits

The **W5** model can be useful for answering questions. The answer should take approximately 90 seconds.

| 70 seconds | **State skill and give an example of it by explaining:**<br><br>• What, Who, When, Where, Why and How<br><br>• What the successful outcome was |
| --- | --- |
| 20 seconds | **Re-state skill and outline benefits transferable to the interviewer's organization** |

For example, in response to the query "What experience do you have organizing projects?" you would determine that the qualification being evaluated is organizational skills. Your Skill/Knowledge/Ability Statement could be, "I have developed excellent organizational skills by working on two major projects. The one I would like to tell you about came to a successful conclusion six months ago." Whatever statement you make must be true! Don't lie or embellish. The illustration you would choose to confirm your statement would be a project that required similar competency to the typical project the prospective employer would want you to organize. Describe the what, who, when, where, why, how, and talk about the successful outcome or what you learned from the experience. As you tell the story, the employer can see or live through the action with you. The next step is the one that most candidates for a position do not include. Tell the interviewer what benefits or competitive advantage you can bring to the position because of that experience. "As part of the team being formed, I would be able to co-ordinate...." The key intention should be to sell yourself by using the story to support your strengths.

## Questions You Can Ask

To supplement information obtained prior to the interview, you need to ask additional questions during the interview. Some questions will arise naturally throughout the interview but it is wise to bring some written questions with you. It shows the interviewer that you prepared for the interview by doing your homework. The questions should be pertinent to the position and show your enthusiasm and knowledge. By asking intelligent, well-thought-out questions, you show the employer you are serious about the organization and need more information. If a question has been answered during the interview, do not ask it again. This will give the impression you are not listening. It is important to write your own questions. To help you do this, refer to the following examples:

• What do you see as the priorities for someone in this position?

**Used with permission from Career Services, University of Waterloo / Source: Career Development eManual www.cdm.uwaterloo.ca**

- Would you be able to describe a typical day on the job?

- What would be a typical first-year assignment?

- What training programs do you have available for your employees?

- What level of responsibility could I expect in this position?

- Is there a typical career path for a person in this position?

- How are employees evaluated and promoted?

- What is a realistic time frame for promotion?

- Does the company have a promotion-from-within policy?

- What are the company's plans for the future?

- What do you see as the greatest threat to the organization?

- What/where are the greatest opportunities for the organization?

- How would you describe your organization's management style and working environment?

- What do you like most about your organization?

- Why is this position available? (Is it a new job or where did the former occupant go?)

## Understanding Verbal and Non-Verbal Communication

Smile when appropriate during the interview. Be enthusiastic and responsive. As you talk about your past and present activities in answer to questions, your passion and energy can be communicated both through the words of your stories and your body language (e.g., an excited tone of voice, leaning forward, nodding your head in agreement). Maintaining eye contact is important; failure to do so may imply a lack of confidence or, worse, cause the employer to question your truthfulness.

Sit comfortably, without slouching. Don't put anything on your lap or in your hands as it will restrict your natural body movement and you may be tempted to 'play' with it. Keep your clipboard, note pad, briefcase, or portfolio on the floor beside your chair for easy retrieval when necessary.

Respond to questions specifically and concisely but give sufficient details to enable the interviewer to evaluate your credentials. Interviewers become frustrated when they have to listen to long rambling answers. Think before you speak. It is quite acceptable to pause before talking in order to organize your thoughts. Avoid verbal fillers such as 'um,' 'ah', 'you know', etc., or repeating the question in order to provide thinking time. Use business language. Avoid slang. Speak clearly.

Prepare in advance to talk about any topic that you are concerned or feel uncomfortable about. If there is something that you don't want an interviewer to inquire about, you can be sure that somehow the interviewer will sense it, and ask.

**Used with permission from Career Services, University of Waterloo / Source: Career Development eManual www.cdm.uwaterloo.ca**

Practice your answer out loud often enough to feel confident when saying it. Maintain poise and self-control. Consider a difficult issue as a learning opportunity, which has made you a better person.

## One-to-One

The most common interview format is one interviewer interviewing one candidate. This is sometimes the first of several interviews. Second and third interviews will usually have a number of interviewers.

## Team / Board Interview With Two or More People

While it is important to have good eye contact with the person who asks you the question, also look at the other persons present periodically in order to include them in your answer. Try to remember each individual's name and use his or her name at some point during the interview.

## General (Group) Interview

This approach is intended to provide applicants with a large amount of information about the organization and the role. The format is used in order to save time and ensure everyone understands the basic facts. This process is usually followed by an individual interview.

## Competitive Group Interview

Many candidates are interviewed at the same time, by one or more interviewers. This type of interview is sometimes utilized when a position being applied for involves team work and the interviewers want to see how you interact in a group setting; when the company wants to see who rises as a leader within the group; or when they have large numbers of people interviewing for several similar roles within the company. It is important to thoughtfully and intelligently contribute, but not monopolize the conversation.

## Structured Interview

The goal of this approach is to eliminate bias and assist the employer in making an objective decision. All candidates are asked the same questions for the employer's ease in evaluating applicants. If there is important information that you have not conveyed by the end of the interview, when asked if you have any questions or anything to add, present your additional qualifications. Usually the interviewer will make written notes of your answers.

## Semi-structured Interview

In a semi-structured interview you have a better opportunity to convey information, as there are fewer pre-determined questions. However, you need to be well prepared and know the points you want to make. You will also be expected to participate in 'carrying' the conversation.

**Used with permission from Career Services, University of Waterloo / Source: Career Development eManual www.cdm.uwaterloo.ca**

## Telephone Interview

Due to the high cost of paying travel expenses for candidates to the employer's location, some first interviews are being conducted by telephone. If the call surprises you and you are not ready for an interview, ask the person to call back in 15 minutes, or arrange another time, which will be mutually convenient. You need time to refresh your memory on the organization and what points you want to make. All advice about interview skills still applies. You just do not have to dress for the occasion. However, you may find that dressing up helps you perform better. Keep your resume and your list of questions to ask in front of you. Have a pen and paper available to note any comments or questions you may have during the interview. It is important to pay attention to the voice tone and tempo. Be sure to change your tone and tempo to demonstrate your interest.

Employers often have a formal rating sheet with predetermined areas such as:

- Neat and clean overall appearance/poise/communicative skills
- Academic/work achievements (learning ability, standards of excellence)
- Special skills (technical, languages, creativity, management, analytic, negotiation)
- Personal characteristics (team player, enthusiastic, dependable, emotionally stable, flexible)
- Self-assessment, goals/ambitions
- Leisure-time activities, balance in life
- Reaction to job/organization
- Potential

## Learning From Your Interview

Evaluate how well you did after each interview. Ask yourself:

- What points did I make that seemed to interest the employer?
- Did I present my qualifications in the best manner possible, giving appropriate examples as evidence?
- Was I able to explain my personal goals, interests and desires?
- Did I emphasize how my skills are related to the role?
- Did I pass up opportunities to sell myself, to demonstrate the work I do and to show how profitably I could do it for both the organization and myself?
- Did I talk too much? Too little?
- Was I too tense? Passive? Aggressive?
- Did I find out enough about the role to make a knowledgeable decision?

**Used with permission from Career Services, University of Waterloo / Source: Career Development eManual www.cdm.uwaterloo.ca**

- What changes can I make for my next interview?

## Tips for Effective Interviewing

1. Get a good night's sleep before your interview.

2. Be punctual. Arrive 15 minutes early to allow yourself time to collect your thoughts. Take the opportunity to observe the working environment. Keep your eyes and ears open. Be friendly with everyone.

3. Try to get the interviewer to describe the position and duties to you early in the interview so that you can relate your background and skills to the particular position.

4. Give **descriptive examples or proof** whenever you can throughout the interview. The true stories you tell about yourself will differentiate you from the other applicants.

5. Watch the interviewer for clues on how the interview is progressing. Is the interviewer's face or body language telling you that your answers are too long, not detailed enough, too boring, etc.? If in doubt, ask the interviewer if more or fewer details are needed.

6. Listen carefully to the question and the way it is phrased. If it can be interpreted in more than one way, and if you are unsure what the interviewer really wants you to discuss, ask for clarification.

7. If the interviewer becomes silent, look for the reason. Has the person momentarily run out of questions? Is the person testing you to see how comfortable you are with silence? Is the interviewer finding your answers too brief and waiting for you to elaborate more in order to get a better sense of who you are?

8. When the interviewer asks about your weaknesses, choose something work-related, but not so serious as to disqualify you. **Briefly** mention one weakness, and then show what you have learned from the experience or what you are doing to change. If pressed for more than one weakness, have another one or two ready to discuss.

9. If you are asked about any negative employment experience (e.g., being fired, trouble with supervisor), don't criticize past employers. Briefly acknowledge any difficulty and say what you have learned or discuss the positive outcome of the situation.

10. Except for co-op scheduled interviews, don't inquire about salary, bonuses or benefits in the initial interview. If you are pressed to give a salary expectation, turn it around to the interviewer and ask what the organization would ordinarily pay a person with your credentials. If you are still pressed, know what salary range would apply to that type of job in that geographic location. Try to obtain this information by speaking to people in the field prior to your interview.

11. Practice in a mock interview with another person. Check for quality of information in your answers, and the positive, non-verbal reinforcement of

your words. By speaking out loud you can "hear" your answers to ensure you cover the topic well. Don't practice so much that you lose your spontaneity and your answers sound rehearsed.

12. If you do not receive a job offer (especially if you felt the "fit" was very good), you may want to contact the interviewer to get feedback on your performance. It could be (1) they hired someone with better qualifications, or (2) you didn't adequately present your qualifications, thereby causing an incorrect assessment of your capability. If the reason is (1), keep going...you'll find the right match! If the reason is (2), learn from this and make the necessary changes in your next interview!

## Your Rights in the Interview

There are clear human rights guidelines for employment interview questions. Applicants for employment may be asked to divulge only information that has relevance to the position applied for. Employers, by law, must focus on gathering relevant information in order to decide if the applicant is able to perform the functions of the position.

Some employers erroneously believe that they have a right to ask any question they choose since they are paying the salary. Others are simply awkward in their technique and an unlawful question results. However, human rights law does not distinguish between the interviewer who is asking questions with the intent to discriminate, and the one who is just curious or inept at interviewing.

There are questions that are appropriate and questions that are illegal. You do not have to answer questions that are illegal. The Ontario Human Rights Code prohibits discrimination in employment on the grounds of:

| | |
|---|---|
| Race | Ancestry |
| Place of origin | Colour |
| Ethnic origin | Citizenship |
| Creed | Sex |
| Sexual orientation | Age |
| Record of offences | Marital status |
| Family status | Disability |

Although it is ultimately the responsibility of the interviewer to know the law, this may not always be the case. It is to your advantage to be informed on the subject.

You've done the reading and know your rights as they pertain to the interview. Now you're in the middle of one and have just been asked what is clearly an illegal question. What should you do? There is no clear-cut answer. Much depends on you.

## Ideas for Handling Illegal Questions

In some cases, you may be able to answer the "hidden" question. Try to think of what information the employer is trying to elicit. Example: "Do you have or plan to have children?" may be a disguise for "Are you going to be able to work overtime?" or "Will you be requesting time off for school holidays/events?" In this example, your answer should convey your willingness to work overtime as required or make alternate child care arrangements.

You may elect to say "Why do you ask?" or "Would you explain how this point is connected to the qualifications for this job?" This may cause the employer to reconsider and/or clarify the question. This may offend some employers, but probably not the majority.

If you feel that you should not answer the question (you shouldn't have to after all) or that you are not interested in working for the company, you may state, "I don't feel obligated to answer that" or "That question is inappropriate". If you choose this option, you will either enlighten (the employer may not realize it is illegal and will be happy that you pointed it out) or offend (the employer may not consider you for the position).

## The Ontario Human Rights Commission

Keep in mind that the vast majority of employers strive to hire the most qualified staff and do so fairly. For employers who don't play by the rules, remember that assistance is available through the Ontario Human Rights Commission office. Contact them. To access the complaint procedure, visit the OHRC Web site at http://www.ohrc.on.ca/

# SAMPLE INTERVIEW QUESTIONS

Typically, a wide variety of questions can be used to gain information about a candidate's job skills. You can use these questions as a guide to help you develop answers to questions that target job skill requirements.

1.  Describe a time when you were faced with problems or stresses that tested your coping skills. What did you do?

2.  Give an example of a time when you could not participate in a discussion or could not finish a task because you did not have enough information.

3.  Give an example of a time when you had to be relatively quick in coming to a decision.

4.  Tell me how your education in Social Sciences helped prepare you for this position.

5.  Tell me about a time when you had to use your verbal communication skills in order to get an important point across to someone else.

6.  Tell me about a job experience in which you had to speak up and tell other people what you thought or felt?

7.  Give me an example of when you felt you were able to motivate your coworkers or subordinates.

8.  Tell me about a specific occasion when you conformed to a policy even though you did not agree with it.

9.  Describe a situation in which you felt it necessary to be very attentive and vigilant to your environment.

10. Give me an example of a time when you used your fact-finding skills to gain information needed to solve a problem; then tell me how you analyzed the information and came to a decision.

11. Give me an example of an important goal you had to set, and tell me about your progress in reaching that goal.

12. Describe the most significant written document, report, or presentation that you have completed.

13. Give me an example of a time when you had to go above and beyond the call of duty in order to a job done.

SOC SCI 2ELO

14. Tell me about a typical day at university and how you planned your day.

15. Describe a time when you had a difficult situation with a peer, co-worker or customer that you were unable to solve.

16. Describe a time at work or school when you made a mistake. What did you learn from this?

17. Tell me about a time when you feel you displayed leadership ability.

18. Describe a situation where you were able to use persuasion to successfully convince someone to see things a different way.

19. Provide an example of a time when you used good judgment and logic in solving a problem.

20. Tell me about a time where you had to set an important goal. Were you successful in achieving this goal?

21. Describe the most creative presentation that you completed.

22. What is the most important skill you have developed through your education?

# WEEK 6

# INFORMATION INTERVIEW

## The Call

Good morning (afternoon). My name is _____. I am a Social Sciences student at McMaster University and am currently in the process of exploring several occupations as part of my career planning.

One occupation that I am particularly interested in is _____. Before I make any decisions about pursuing a career in this area, I would like to meet with you to get some advice and information regarding the occupation. It should only take about _____ minutes of your time. If this is possible, when would be a convenient time for you?

## The Information Interview

*Before the Interview:*

- Do your research before. Find out as much as you can about the occupation/field and the company you will be meeting with.
- Prepare questions to ask...and be prepared to answer questions they may have about you and your interests in the field.
- Confirm your appointment. When will it be? With whom?

*During the Interview:*

- Introduce yourself and thank them for meeting with you.
- Respect the length of the appointment you set.
- Show interest and enthusiasm.
- Ask for referrals to others they know or other resources they would recommend.
- If appropriate ask for a tour of the office/facility (it will help you visualize what the work environment may be like).
- Ask if you can approach them again should you have any questions at a later date.
- Ask for their business card.

*After the Interview:*

- Follow up on all contacts or recommendations that were made.
- Update the contacts on how their recommendations may have helped.
- Send a thank you letter/email.
- Add this person to your networking list.

# SAMPLE THANK YOU LETTER

The following is a sample of a typical 'Thank You' letter. Please note that this is only one example and that there are many other ways to compose this type of letter. The important thing is that you acknowledge and thank the person who granted you the information interview.

---

September 10, 2017


Ms Janet McMaster
Senior Manager
Excel and Associates
125 Hildebrant Street
Anytown, Ontario
A1F 3P3


Dear Janet,

Thank you for allowing me to visit with you and share in your career experience. I discovered much about the _____ field and feel that my time with you has assisted me in making goals for my own career.

I appreciate your time and effort and wish you the best of luck for your future.

Sincerely,



Joe Smith